Mosby's Medical Assisting Video Workbook

Neila J. Burrows, CMA-A

Publisher: David T. Culverwell
Acquisitions Editor: Eric M. Duchinsky
Senior Developmental Editor: Cecilia F. Reilly
Assistant Editor: Christine H. Ambrose
Editorial Assistant: Kenneth E. Queen II
Book Design and Production: Barbara Campbell
Cover Design: Mastercraft Graphics

The following artwork was borrowed from *Clinical Procedures for Medical Assistants* 3/E by Sharron M. Zakus, St. Louis, 1995, Mosby:

Un-numbered figures on pages 3, 25, 48, 65, 83, 103, 127, 149, 169, 187, 203, and 221.

Figures 4-1, 5-1, 5-2, 5-4, 7-1, 7-2 A and B, 7-3, 7-4, 8-1, 8-2, 8-3, 8-4, 9-1, 9-2 A through C, 9-3, 10-1 A through H, 10-2, and 11-3.

Printed in the United States of America

Composition by: Barbara Campbell

Printing/Binding by:

Mosby-Year Book, Inc.
11830 Westline Industrial Drive
St. Louis, Missouri 63146

International Standard Book Number 0-8151-0518-5

95 96 97 98 99 2000 / 9 8 7 6 5 4 3 2 1

Contents

Introduction

This workbook is written to accompany Mosby's Medical Assistant Video Series. It is designed to help you review and master the concepts and techniques presented in the videos. The medical assistant's primary responsibilities are technical in nature. Enhancement of each subject adds interest and increases your understanding of current activities in the healthcare setting.

The workbook is organized as follows:

Historical Highlights

Historical Highlights are vignettes, brief sketches of medicine's past, to encourage you to explore the past and to creatively look toward the future.

Evaluation

Vocabulary presents selected terms from the video and supplemental language to expand the medical assistant's skill in medical terminology.

Student Activities are a wide assortment of research and reference projects designed to acquaint you with the ever increasing boundaries of medical assisting.

Discussion Topics revolve around current issues. They encourage open discussion of different healthcare issues as well as problems and concerns facing the medical assistant.

Review and Rationale is a series of "why" questions. If each question is transposed into a statement, it represents a fact presented in the video for review. By answering the "why" question, you demonstrate not only your knowledge of the concept but the rationale supporting it.

Performance Test and Checklist is a final demonstration of skill level attained by completing the video and workbook exercises. Performance must be demonstrated within acceptable time frames and proficiency observed and documented by your instructor.

Evaluation consists of multiple choice and true/false questions as a final demonstration of your level of proficiency on the material presented in the video.

Word Puzzles are presented for additional practice in vocabulary building.

Answer Key

For reinforcement, an end-of-the-chapter answer key is provided. In addition to the answers to quizzes and evaluations, it includes suggestions and sources for many of the *Student Activities* and *Discussion Topics.* However, you are encouraged to pursue the research projects first before consulting the key. You will get more out of researching the answers yourself and it will give you excellent resources for the future. Answer as many of the questions as you can based on your knowledge from watching the videos. Compare your answers with the answer key; if you are missing an answer or have an error, go back and review the video. Do not erase your incorrect answer. Instead, use a different color ink to write the correct answer. You will have a record of what you need to pay particular attention to when you review the video.

— *Neila J. Burrows, CMA-A*

HISTORICAL HIGHLIGHTS

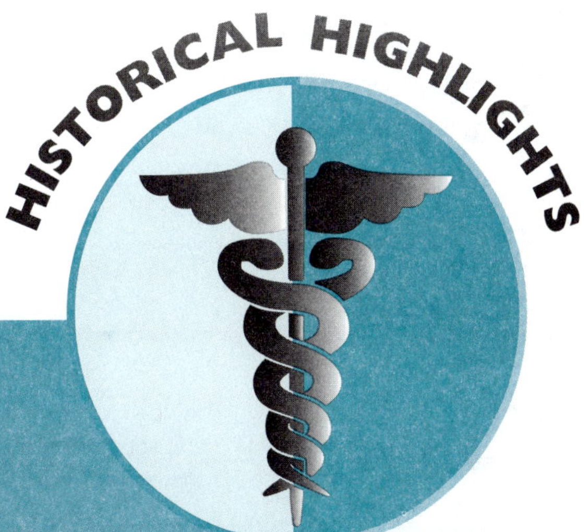

According to Mosby's Medical, Nursing, & Allied Health Dictionary, the Latin term caduceus means the wand of the god Hermes or Mercury. It is represented as a staff with two serpents coiled around it. This symbol is used as the medical insignia of certain groups such as the U.S. Army Medical Corps. Even though it is sometimes used to symbolize the medical profession, the staff of Aesculapius (the Roman god of medicine) is considered to be the more appropriate symbol.

Aesculapius is the son of Apollo and the nymph Coronis. His staff or crude stick has a snake wound around it. Snakes were sacred to Aesculapius because it was believed that they had the power to renew their youth by shedding their old skin and growing a new one. The staff of Aesculapius is used to signify the art of healing and is used by many medical organizations.

This icon has been chosen to precede each section of Historical Highlights to represent your chosen profession.

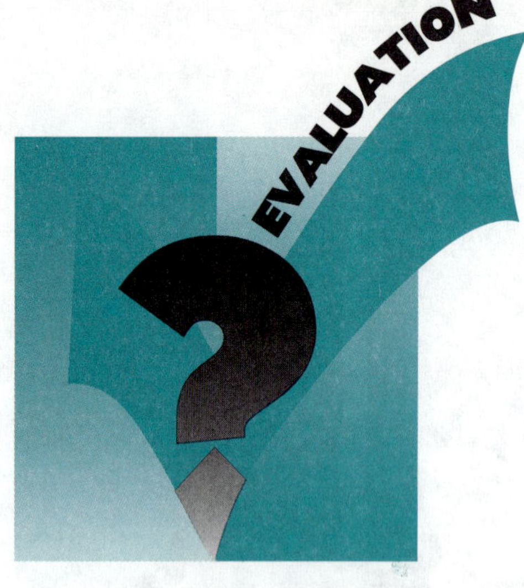

Vocabulary

Write the letter of each term on the line of its matching definition at the right.

a. sublingual pocket

b. oral thermometer

c. pulse

d. rectal thermometer

e. tympanic thermometer

f. temperature

g. respiration

h. blood pressure

i. systole

j. diastole

k. TPR

l. sphygmomanometer

m. brachial pulse

n. hypotension

o. exhalation

1. _______ the period when the heart muscle contracts and squeezes blood out of the heart and to the body

2. _______ first three vital signs

3. _______ the act of inhalation

4. _______ beat of the heart as felt through the walls of the arteries

5. _______ result of the balance between heat produced and heat lost by the body

6. _______ the amount of force exerted by the blood against the walls of the blood vessels

7. _______ the beat of the heart as felt through the walls of the arteries in the arm

8. _______ blood pressure under 90 mg Hb with a diastolic pressure in proportion

9. _______ device used to measure pulse

10. _______ thermometer used to record the most accurate temperature

11. _______ red-collared electronic probe

12. _______ the act of breathing air out of the lungs

13. _______ device used to record temperature via the mouth

14. _______ the period when the heart muscle relaxes and fills with blood

15. _______ area beneath the tongue used for placement of a thermometer

Student Activity

1. Several techniques are used in the physical examination of patients. These terms can be applied when measuring vital signs. Using a medical dictionary, define the following terms and be prepared to use them appropriately in the Discussion Topics:

a. auscultation
b. inspection
c. manipulation
d. palpation
e. percussion

Discussion Topics

1. The medical assistant has just completed taking a patient's temperature using an electronic thermometer and replaced the probe into its holder before writing the temperature down. Now she realizes she has forgotten the temperature. How can she obtain the patient's temperature?

2. The medical assistant has failed to instruct the patient to remain still while the rectal thermometer is in place. What are the potential consequences of such neglect?

3. The medical assistant used her thumb to take the patient's pulse. Was there any reason not to use the thumb? If so, explain which fingers should be used and why.

4. Discuss why you should not explain to a patient when you take respirations.

5. Explain the rationale about blood pressure falling only two to three millimeters of mercury at a time.

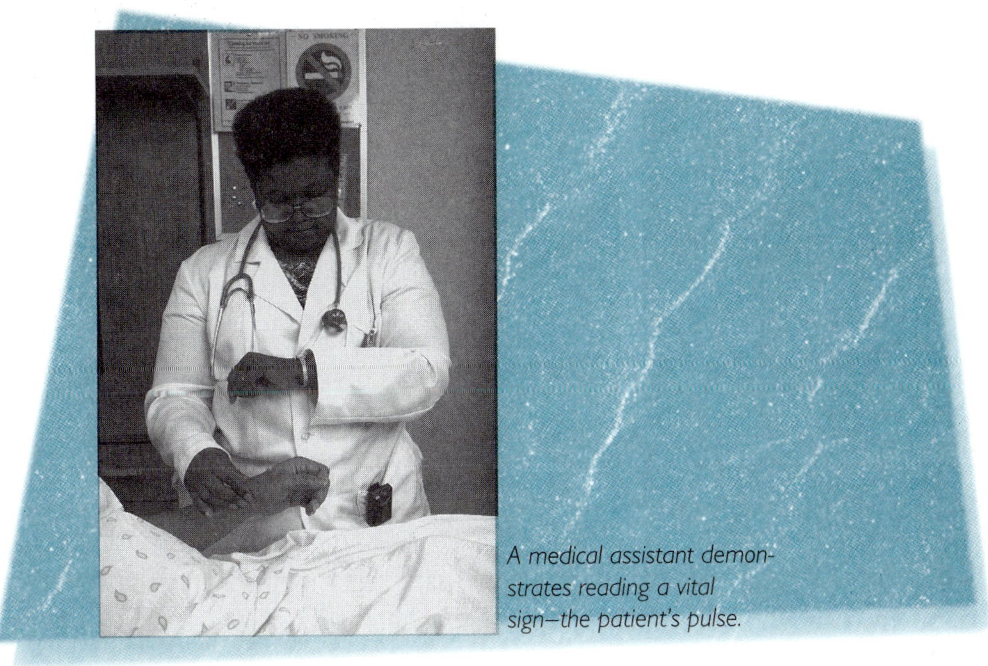

A medical assistant demonstrates reading a vital sign—the patient's pulse.

Review and Rationale

Answer the following questions in the space provided.

1. Why are thermometers calibrated in Fahrenheit and Centigrade degrees?

____

____

____

2. Why should a glass thermometer be read using adequate lighting?

____

____

____

3. Why is it important that you write down the temperature before replacing the probe into its holder?

____

____

____

4. Why is it important to note an irregular pulse rate?

____

____

____

5. Why should you press gently with your first three fingers below the person's thumb on the inner wrist when taking a pulse?

____

____

____

6. Why is it not possible to take a rectal temperature, pulse, and respirations at the same
time?

____

____

____

7. Why is it extremely important that blood pressure be measured accurately?

____

____

____

8. Why sit the patient on the examining table following orthostatic blood pressure reading?

____

____

____

Performance Test

In a skills laboratory, a simulation of a job-like environment, the medical assistant student
must demonstrate knowledge and skill in performing the following procedures without reference to source materials. For these activities you will need a watch with a second hand,
oral, rectal, axillary, and tympanic thermometers; a stethoscope; sphygmomanometer; alcohol sponges; containers for used thermometers; various individuals to play the role of a
patient; and paper and pen. Time limits and number of patients to be tested for each procedure are to be assigned by the instructor.

Given an ambulatory patient and the appropriate equipment and supplies, obtain and
record accurately:*

   1. oral temperature using a glass thermometer

   2. oral temperature using an electronic thermometer

   3. axillary temperature

   4. rectal temperature (a model may be used for this procedure)

   5. radial pulse

6. apical pulse

7. respiratory rate

8. blood pressure using brachial artery

9. orthostatic blood pressure

Results obtained for the pulse rates and the respiratory rates are acceptable if within two beats or respirations as determined and recorded by the instructor. Results for blood pressure readings are acceptable if within 2 to 4 mm. Hg., as determined and recorded by the instructor. The student is expected to attain proficiency in these procedures before progressing to other videos.

Performance Checklist

DIRECTIONS: The following checklist will be used to evaluate your performance of each procedure.

Checklist 1-1: Taking oral temperature using a glass thermometer.

Checklist	S or NA	U	NO	Comment
1. Identify yourself and the patient and explain the procedure.				
2. Wash hands.				
3. Assemble equipment.				
4. Position patient and explain procedure.				
5. Remove the clean thermometer from the storage container and rinse it with cold running water. Wipe dry from the stem downward to the bulb with a tissue or cotton square and discard material used.				
6. With a firm hold on the end of the thermometer, shake the mercury down to 96 degrees Fahrenheit or below.				
7. Place the thermometer to the side of the mouth, well under the patient's tongue and instruct patient to keep lips closed and to breath through the mouth. Leave the thermometer in place for three minutes.				
8. Remove the thermometer and wipe it from the top toward the bulb.				
9. Read the thermometer and record the temperature at once, noting that it was an oral temperature.				
10. Shake down the mercury to 96 degrees and place the thermometer in the container for used oral thermometers.				
11. Wash your hands.				

*S or NA = satisfactory or not applicable; U = unsatisfactory; NO = not observed

Checklist 1-2: Taking oral temperature with an electronic thermometer.

Checklist	S or NA	U	NO	Comment
1. Identify yourself and the patient and explain the procedure.				
2. Wash hands.				
3. Assemble equipment.				
4. Position patient and explain procedure.				
5. Remove the probe from the probe holder and insert it firmly into an unused plastic cover.				
6. Check the digital display window for the temperature.				
7. Place the probe slowly into the sublingual pocket of the mouth holding the probe in place.				
8. Watch the thermometer display.				
9. Gently remove the probe from the mouth, eject the cover into the infectious waste bag and read the temperature in the digital display window.				
10. Write the temperature down as T=, indicating that it was taken orally.				
11. Wash your hands.				

*S or NA = satisfactory or not applicable; U = unsatisfactory; NO = not observed

Checklist 1-3: Taking axillary using oral thermometer.

Checklist	S or NA	U	NO	Comment
1. Identify yourself and the patient and explain the procedure.				
2. Wash hands.				
3. Assemble equipment.				
4. Position patient and explain procedure.				
5. Expose the person's underarm and blot the axillary region dry with a tissue or a cotton square.				
6. Place the bulb end of the thermometer in the hollow of the axillary region with the end of the thermometer slanting toward the patient's chest.				
7. Ask the patient to cross his arm over his chest or to hold his opposite shoulder.				
8. Leave the thermometer in place for five to ten minutes.				
9. Remove and wipe the thermometer from the top toward the bulb with a tissue, and read it.				
10. Record the reading at once as T=, noting that an axillary temperature was taken.				
11. Wash your hands.				

*S or NA = satisfactory or not applicable; U = unsatisfactory; NO = not observed

Checklist 1-4: Taking rectal temperature using rectal thermometer.

Checklist	S or NA	U	NO	Comment
1. Identify yourself and the patient and explain the procedure.				
2. Wash hands.				
3. Assemble equipment.				
4. Position patient and explain procedure.				
5. Ask patient to remove only the clothing necessary to provide access to the buttocks area.				
6. Provide a drape for comfort and privacy.				
7. Assist the patient to turn on his side, facing away from you.				
8. Bend the upper leg to make it easier for the patient to remain in the side-lying position.				
9. Put on gloves.				
10. Apply plastic sheath to thermometer, if applicable.				
11. Apply lubricant to the thermometer with a tissue.				
12. Turn back the patient's drape, and separate the buttocks to expose the anus.				
13. Gently insert the thermometer one inch into the anal canal while instructing patient to remain still.				
14. Hold the thermometer in place for three to five minutes.				
15. Remove the thermometer and wipe the person's anal area with a tissue.				
16. Take off the sheath covering, if used.				
17. Wipe the thermometer from the top toward the bulb and read the temperature accurately.				
18. Record the reading as T=, noting that a rectal temperature was taken.				
19. Shake the mercury down to 96 degrees Fahrenheit.				
20. Place the thermometer in the container for used rectal thermometers.				
21. Dispose of gloves and wash hands.				
22. Provide for patient's comfort.				
23. Assist patient with dressing, if necessary.				

*S or NA = satisfactory or not applicable; U = unsatisfactory; NO = not observed

Checklist 1-5: Recording the radial pulse.

Checklist	S or NA	U	NO	Comment
1. Identify yourself and the patient and explain the procedure.				
2. Wash your hands.				
3. Assemble equipment.				
4. Position patient and explain procedure.				
5. Find the radial pulse using correct technique and positioning.				
6. Count for one full minute.				
7. Note rate, rhythm, volume, and condition. Report any pulse more or less than acceptable.				
8. Record pulse as P= or pulse =.				

*S or NA = satisfactory or not applicable; U = unsatisfactory; NO = not observed

Checklist 1-6: Recording the apical pulse.

Checklist	S or NA	U	NO	Comment
1. Identify yourself and the patient and explain the procedure.				
2. Wash your hands.				
3. Assemble equipment.				
4. Position patient and explain procedure.				
5. Clean the earpieces and the chestpiece of the stethoscope with an alcohol sponge.				
6. Place the stethoscope diaphragm over the apex of the heart and count the number of heartbeats for one minute.				
7. Record the results as P=, indicating an apical pulse was taken.				
8. Wipe the ear pieces and diaphragm of the stethoscope with an alcohol sponge and return it to the proper storage area.				
9. Wash hands.				

*S or NA = satisfactory or not applicable; U = unsatisfactory; NO = not observed

Checklist 1-7: Recording respiration.

Checklist	S or NA	U	NO	Comment
1. Identify yourself and the patient but do not explain the procedure.				
2. Wash your hands.				
3. Assemble equipment.				
4. Place your fingers on the patient's wrist as though taking a pulse.				
5. Count respirations for one full minute.				
6. Record the rate as R=. Note any pain associated with breathing.				

*S or NA = satisfactory or not applicable; U = unsatisfactory; NO = not observed

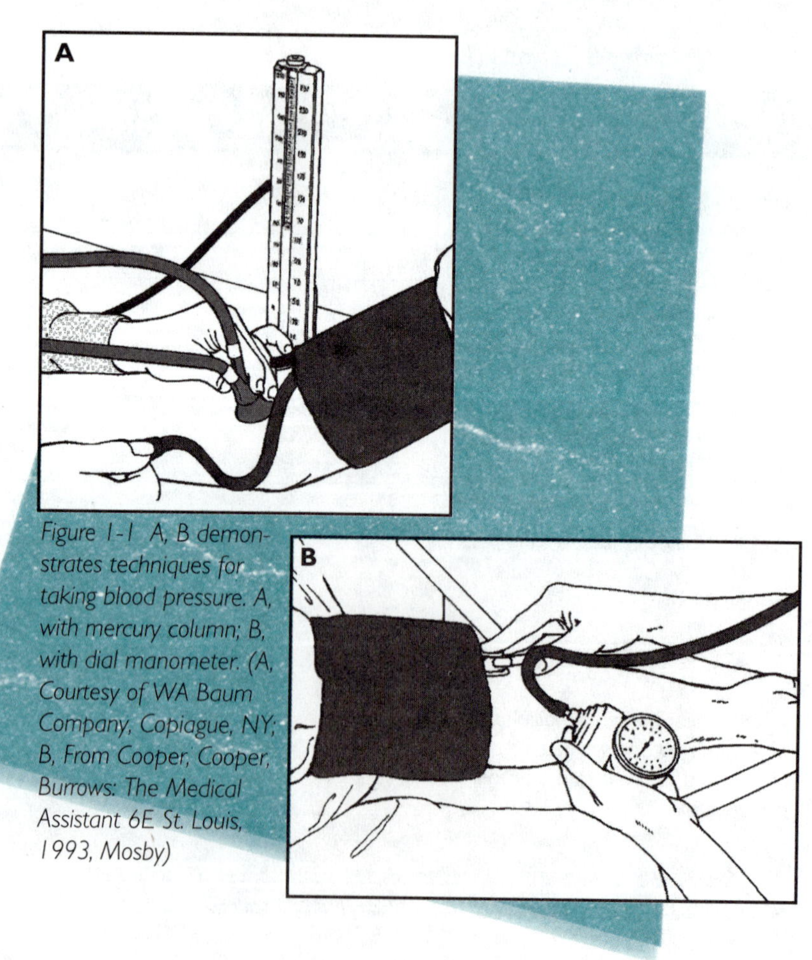

Figure 1-1 A, B demonstrates techniques for taking blood pressure. A, with mercury column; B, with dial manometer. (A, Courtesy of WA Baum Company, Copiague, NY; B, From Cooper, Cooper, Burrows: The Medical Assistant 6E St. Louis, 1993, Mosby)

Checklist 1-8: Measure blood pressure of brachial pulse in sitting position.

Checklist	S or NA	U	NO	Comment
1. Identify yourself and the patient and explain the procedure.				
2. Wash your hands.				
3. Assemble equipment.				
4. Clean the earpieces and the chestpiece of the stethoscope with an alcohol sponge.				
5. Help the patient to a comfortable sitting position.				
6. The arm selected for blood pressure measurement should be extended and supported.				
7. Place the sphygmomanometer at your eye level.				
8. Expose the patient's arm well above the elbow and apply the cuff with the arrows pointing over the brachial artery one to two inches above the antecubital space.				
9. Wrap the remainder of the cuff snugly around the arm, overlapping one end over the other.				
10. Find the strongest point of the patient's brachial pulse by palpating with fingers at the bend of the elbow.				
11. Adjust the earpieces of the stethoscope in your ears and place the diaphragm or bells directly over the stongest brachial pulsation. Hold chestpiece in place. (See Figure 1-1, A, B)				
12. Close the air valve in clockwise direction.				
13. Pump air into the cuff rapidly until the level of mercury or the aneroid needle reads 180 to 200 mm. of Hg.				
14. Release the cuff air by turning the air valve slowly counter clockwise. (Pressure should not exceed 2-3 mm. of Hg. at a time.)				

*S or NA = satisfactory or not applicable; U = unsatisfactory; NO = not observed

Continued on next page

Continued from previous page

Checklist 1-8: Measure blood pressure of brachial pulse in sitting position

Checklist	S or NA	U	NO	Comment
15. Listening carefully, read the systolic pressure distinct while continuing to slowly deflate the cuff. Continue to deflate the cuff until the sound disappears. Write the blood pressure reading down on paper as a mathematical fraction indicating where the sound disappears.				
16. Remove the cuff from the patient's arm and provide for his comfort.				
17. Return the equipment to its designated area.				
18. Clean the earpieces and the diaphragm of the stethoscope with an alcohol sponge.				
19. Notify the physician of abnormally high or low findings.				

*S or NA = satisfactory or not applicable; U = unsatisfactory; NO = not observed

Checklist 1-9: Orthostatic blood pressure

Checklist	S or NA	U	NO	Comment
1. Identify yourself and the patient and explain the procedure.				
2. Watch for any signs of dizziness or weakness.				
3. Assemble equipment.				
4. Request patient to lie down for five minutes.				
5. Take blood pressure and an apical pulse.				
6. Record this reading, indicating that it was taken in a lying position.				
7. Ask patient to sit up at a ninety degree angle and take a blood pressure and apical pulse immediately.				
8. Ask patient how he feels.				
9. Record this reading, indicating a sitting position.				
10. Request the patient to stand at the side of the examining table.				
11. Question him about any feelings of dizziness or weakness.				
12. Take the blood pressure and apical pulse immediately.				
13. After reading the measurement, sit the patient on the examining table and assure his comfort and safety.				
14. Record this reading as a mathematical fraction, indicating standing position.				

*S or NA = satisfactory or not applicable; U = unsatisfactory; NO = not observed

Multiple Choice

From the options listed under each question or statement, select the correct answer or answers. Write the corresponding letter or letters in the answer space.

1. Blood pressure is influenced by: ________
   a. the strength of the heart's contractions
   b. amount of blood pumped with each heart beat
   c. the blood's thickness or thinness
   d. the ease with which the blood is able to flow through the body
   e. all of the above

2. The volume of the pulse refers to the strength of the pulsations and may be described as: ________
   a. soft or elastic
   b. regular or irregular
   c. full, bounding, weak, thready, hard or soft
   d. none of the above

3. Body sites where the pulse can most easily be felt are: ________
   a. carotid, brachial, radial, popliteal, and pedal
   b. dorsalis pedis, radial, and carotid
   c. pedal, dorsalis pedis, brachial, and radial
   d. popliteal, brachial, carotid, and radial

4. Rate means: ________
   a. time interval between each beat
   b. number of pulsations or beats in a given minute
   c. rise and fall of the chest
   d. amount of air inhaled and exhaled

5. Which of the following factors can affect the blood pressure? ________
   a. exercise
   b. stress
   c. smoking
   d. increased weight
   e. medications or certain disease
   f. all of the above.

6. Glass thermometers are calibrated in: ________
   a. degrees
   b. fahrenheit
   c. metric
   d. centigrade
   e. b and d
   f. none of the above

7. When taking an oral temperature, leave the thermometer in place for __________ minutes:

    a. 5

    b. 2

    c. 3

    d. 1

8. An example of a water-soluble lubricant used when taking a rectal temperature is which of the following: ________

    a. K-Y jelly

    b. vaseline

    c. A&D ointment

    d. petroleum jelly

9. Which of the following methods of temperature recording is most accurate? ________

    a. oral

    b. rectal

    c. tympanic

    d. axillary

10. Which of the following is the 2nd vital sign? ________

    a. blood pressure

    b. temperature

    c. respiration

    d. pulse

True or False

Determine whether each of the following statements is true or false. Check the box marked T or F at the left of the statement.

T   F

☐ ☐ 1. Hypertension is indicated by a systolic pressure reading over 160 mm of Hg and a diastolic pressure over 90 mm. Hg.

☐ ☐ 2. Depth is described as regular or irregular.

☐ ☐ 3. Rhythm is described as shallow or deep.

☐ ☐ 4. Blood pressure is measured in number of millimeters of mercury.

☐ ☐ 5. Rate refers to the number of respirations per minute.

T F

☐ ☐ 6. When measuring a person's blood pressure, there are two readings you need to take—systolic and diastolic.

☐ ☐ 7. Blood pressure is recorded and discussed as the systolic pressure over the diastolic pressure.

☐ ☐ 8. A regular pulse rate has no interval between pulsations.

☐ ☐ 9. A normal arterial wall is described as hard or knotty.

☐ ☐ 10. An oral thermometer has a red end.

Word Puzzle

Circle the following medical terms related to vital signs.

radial	rate	tongue	oral
ear	blood	mercury	rectal
brachial	diastole	manipulation	apical
temperature	orthostatic	stethoscope	thermometer
auscultate	inspection	hypotension	sphygmomanometer

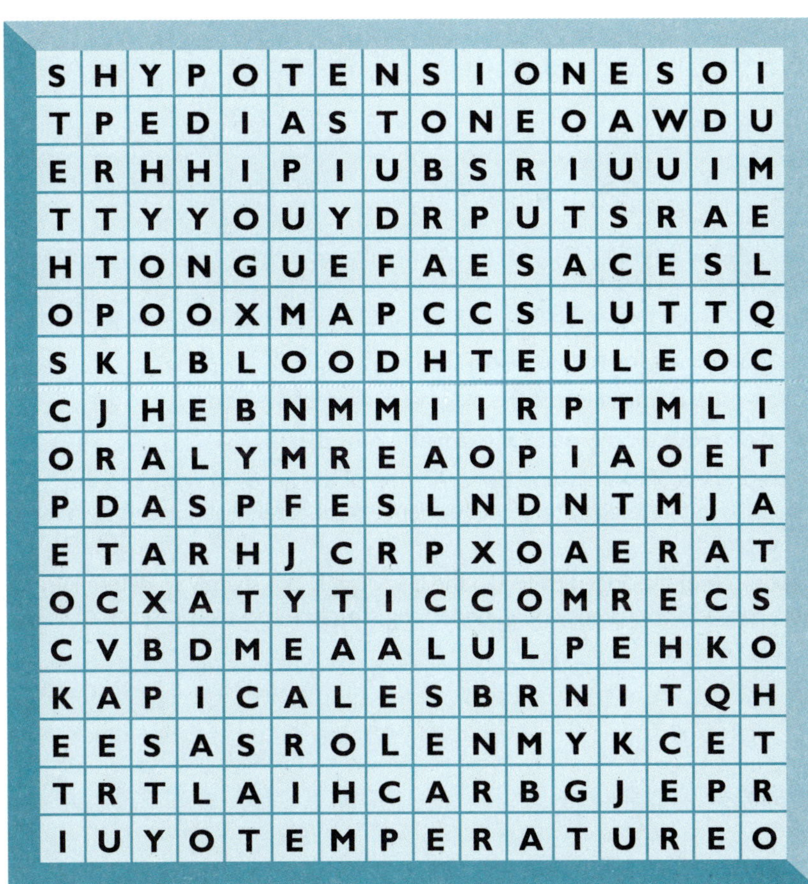

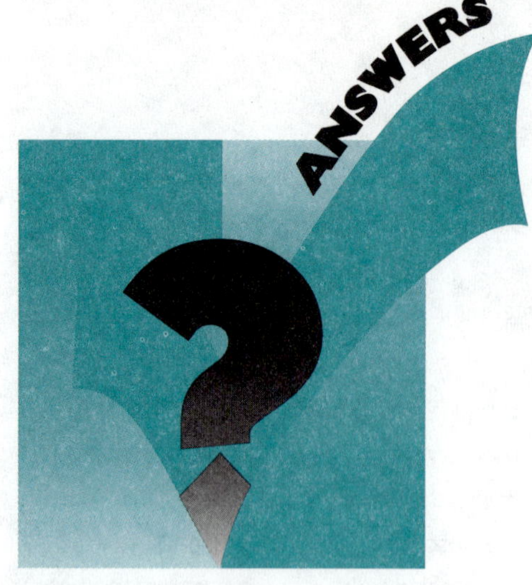

Vocabulary

1. i	4. c	7. m	10. e	13. b
2. k	5. f	8. n	11. d	14. j
3. g	6. h	9. l	12. o	15. a

Student Activity

1. a. auscultation-listening for sounds within the body
    b. inspection-visual examination of the external surface of the body
    c. manipulation-move a body part for examination or therapy
    d. palpation-process of examination by application of the hands or fingers to the external surface of the body to detect evidence of disease or abnormalities in the various organs
    e. percussion-use of the fingertips to tap the body lightly but sharply to determine position, size, and consistency of an underlying structure and the presence of fluid or pus in a cavity

Discussion Topics

1. Once the probe has been replaced into its holder the temperature is erased. Therefore, the medical assistant should take the temperature a second time.

2. Movement may cause the thermometer to slip out of or go further into the rectum.

3. Never use your thumb to take a pulse, as your thumb's pulse may be confused with the patient's. Use index, middle, and third fingers.

4. Do not explain the procedure as the patient's consciousness of being watched will cause him to change his respiration rate.

5. Pressure should only fall two to three millimeters of mercury at a time because rapid deflation of the cuff will cause you to miss the exact blood pressure reading.

Review and Rationale

1. As the metric system is being used more frequently, you should know how to convert Fahrenheit degrees to Centigrade.

2. Be sure that the lighting is adequate when reading a glass thermometer so that you can see the line better by changing the direction of your light source.

3. It is important that you write down the temperature before replacing the probe into its holder because replacing the probe will erase the temperature display.

4. It is important to note an irregular pulse rate showing frequent skipping pulsations or pulsations unequal in length so the physician can be alerted to important signs of heart disease.

5. Excessive pressure on the artery prevents the pulse from being felt.

6. It is not possible to take the patient's rectal temperature at the same time you are taking pulse and respirations because of the patient's position.

7. Blood pressure measurements provide the physician with valuable information about the patient's cardiovascular system.

8. Sit the patient on the examining table and assure his comfort and safety following orthostatic blood pressure reading.

Multiple Choice

1. e	3. a	5. f	7. c	9. c
2. c	4. b	6. e	8. a	10. d

True or False

1. T	3. F	5. T	7. T	9. F
2. F	4. T	6. T	8. F	10. F

Word Puzzle

```
S H Y P O T E N S I O N E S O I
T P E D I A S T O N E O A W D U
E R H H I P I U B S R I U U I M
T T Y Y O U Y D R P U T S R A E
H T O N G U E F A E S A C E S L
O P O O X M A P C C S L U T T Q
S K L B L O O D H T E U L E O C
C J H E B N M M I I R P T M L I
O R A L Y M R E A O P I A O E T
P D A S P F E S L N D N T M J A
E T A R H J C R P X O A E R A T
O C X A T Y T I C C O M R E C S
C V B D M E A A L U L P E H K O
K A P I C A L E S B R N I T Q H
E E S A S R O L E N M Y K C E T
T R T L A I H C A R B G J E P R
I U Y O T E M P E R A T U R E O
```

HISTORICAL HIGHLIGHTS

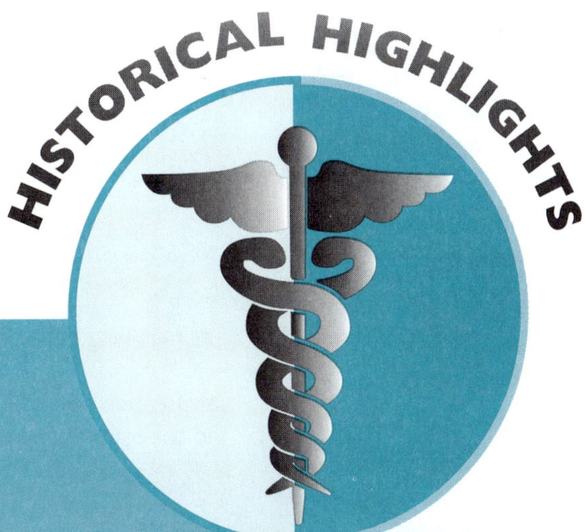

Ever since the dawn of civilization man has used drugs and poisons and he experimented with plant, mineral, and animal substances for the treatment of illness. Over the course of centuries, folklore about the curative virtues of such products developed. The earliest known prescriptions are from Egypt and the most important of those are the so-called Ebers papyrus discovered in Thebes. The Ebers papyrus dates from the time of Moses, 1550 B.C. They deal primarily with prescriptions containing oil, yeast, turpentine, castor oil, aloe, opium, peppermint, cassia, caraway, coriander, and honey, to name just a few.

After the death of Aesculapius, temples were built in many parts of Greece and a secret society of the Aesclepiades (those who claimed to be true descendants of the mythological Aesculapius) became repositories of medical and pharmaceutical lore. Whenever therapeutic treatments were discovered, the prescriptions were engraved on the pillars, door-posts, or walls of the temple.

Over 4000 years ago, King Hammurabi of Babylonia codified the laws of human behavior. These included severe penalties for a physician who did not cure, such as cutting off the physician's hands. Although this ancient punishment seems severe by contemporary judgment, it should remind all health-care workers that the primary consideration is to do patients no harm.

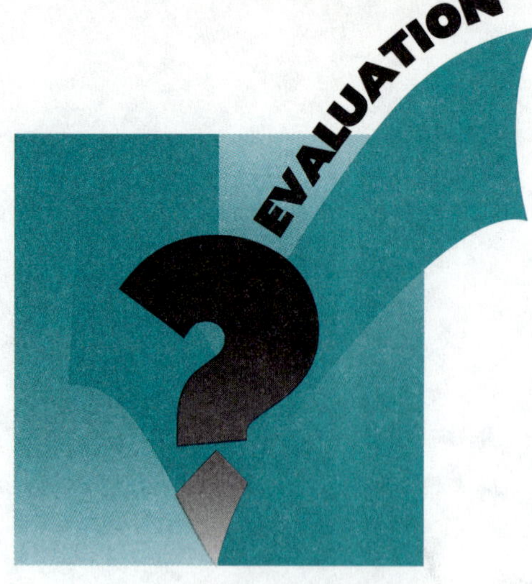

Vocabulary

Write the letter of each term on the line of its matching definition at the right.

a. history

b. physical examination

c. ROS

d. ophthalmoscope

e. neurological pin wheel

f. percussion hammer

g. stethoscope

h. proctoscope

i. vaginal speculum

j. forceps

k. lithotomy

l. dorsal recumbent

m. knee-chest

n. Sims'

o. supine

1. _____ patient kneels on table, keeping buttocks elevated and back straight, head turned to one side

2. _____ instrument used to examine the rectum

3. _____ a sharp-pointed object to elicit pain stimuli

4. _____ pincers for holding, seizing, or extracting

5. _____ position in which patient lies on back with legs separated and knees flexed and feet are supported in stirrups

6. _____ a series of questions and answers about the patient's chief complaint, past, present and family illnesses, social and occupational status

7. _____ a device used for diagnosis consisting of a rubber or metal head used to tap the body lightly but sharply

8. _____ systematic approach to examination of each body system

9. _____ instrument with two opposing portions that after being inserted in a canal can be pushed apart

10. _____ position in which soles of feet are placed flat on table

11. _____ patient lies on table onto the left side and chest, buttocks near edge of table, left leg slightly flexed, right leg sharply flexed

12. _____ instrument used to hear sounds produced in the body

13. _____ a thorough examination of the patient from head to toe

14. _____ patient lies flat on his back, arms placed at sides

15. _____ an instrument for examining interior of the eye

Student Activities

1. Developing interviewing techniques takes practice. Compile a list of questions to ask patients about the following categories:

a. reasons for contacting the doctor
b. biographical data
c. current health status
d. past health history
e. family history
f. social history
g. occupational history

2. Direct and indirect techniques encourage patients to verbalize their feelings and help the medical assistant gather data which will help the physician diagnose problems. Questions directed to focus patients to explain what they are experiencing is direct technique. For example, "Tell me more about your pain"; "How old are you?"; or "Have you experienced this before?" Indirect technique allows the patient to select or elaborate on a subject. For example, "I'm listening, please continue;" or "Go on." Compile a list of both direct and indirect questions or comments that open the dialogue between medical assistant and patient when taking the medical history.

3. Current health status is a general impression of the patient's present state of health. It should include information about the patient's daily life style and activities, including diet and elimination; personal hygiene; use of alcohol and drugs; recreation and exercise; and sleep. List five questions which would elicit information about each of these categories.

4. Obtain identifying information and the medical history from a patient. Use the preprinted medical record forms (Figure 2-1 A–C) to complete the medical history for each of the following:

a. an adult male or female between 30–50 years of age,
b. an elderly male or female over 65 years of age, and
c. a child or adolescent less than 15 years of age.

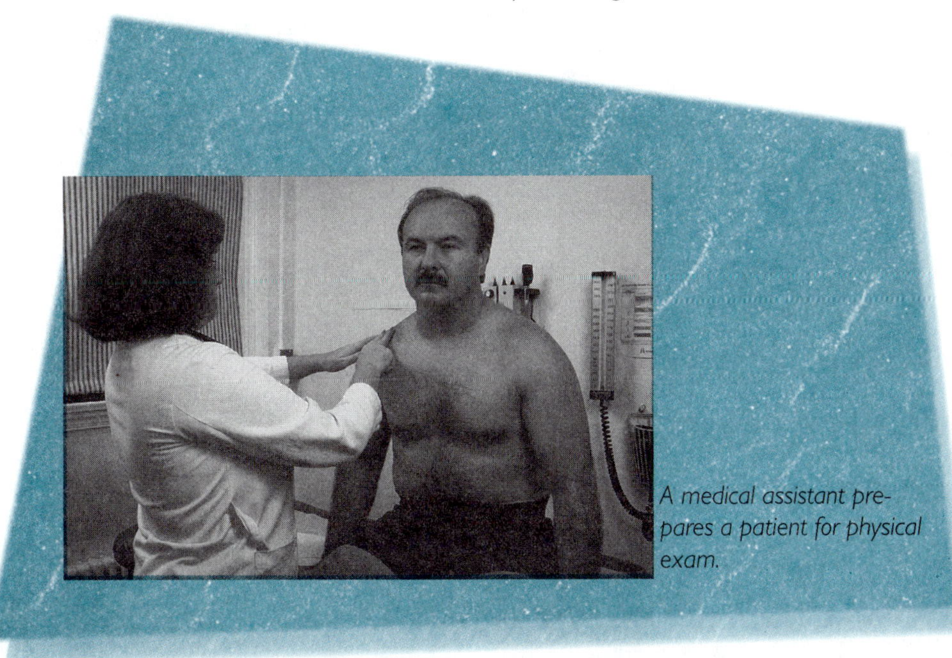

A medical assistant prepares a patient for physical exam.

Figure 2-1A   **MEDICAL RECORD**

NAME	AGE SEX S M D W
ADDRESS	PHONE DATE
Sponsor	address
OCCUPATION	REF BY ACKN

CHIEF COMPLAINT

PRESENT ILLNESS

FAMILY HISTORY	*URINARY TRACT*
MOTHER FATHER	NOCTURIA FREQUENCY
BROTHERS	PAIN BURNING
SISTERS	BLEEDING INFECTION
TB DIAB MALIG	INCONTINENCE
HT DIS NEPH EPILIP	GENITAL TRACT
PSYCH	AGE AT MENST TYPE PERIOD
PAST HISTORY — GENERAL HEALTH	INTERMEN BLEEDING
	AMENORRHEA DYSMENORRHEA
CHILDHOOD DISEASES	VAG DISCH IRRITATION
SC FEV RHEUM FEV ALLERGY	PAINFUL PERIOD
OTHER	L M P
USUAL WEIGHT	CHILDREN L D SB
ACCIDENTS	MARRIED YRS. YOUNGEST CHILD
HABITS COFFEE TOBACCO ALCOHOL	NEURO-MUSCULAR
REVIEW OF SYSTEMS	STRENGTH NERVOUSNESS
E E N T — EYES	SLEEP WORRY
EARS	MUSCULAR PAIN
NOSE	JOINT PAIN
THROAT	ABNORMAL SENSATIONS
NECK	DEFORMITIES
BREASTS	
HEART—LUNGS	**OPERATIONS**
PAIN COUGH	
BLEEDING DYSPNEA	
IRREG EDEMA	
GASTRO-INTESTINAL	**TREATMENTS**
APPETITE DIET	
INDIGESTION PAIN	
NAUSEA VOMITING	
JAUNDICE BLEEDING	**COMMENT**
BOWEL HABITS	
HEMORRHOIDS	
PAIN WITH STOOL ITCHING	
OTHER	

PHYSICAL EXAMINATION

WT	HT	TEMP	BLOOD PRESSURE	PULSE	RESP

GENERAL APPEARANCE

SKIN—SCALP

BLOOD VESSELS

EYES	EARS	NOSE

MOUTH—TEETH

THROAT

NECK

BREASTS

HEART

LUNGS

RIBS

SPINE

ABDOMEN

HERNIA

EXTREMITIES

REFLEXES

LYMPH NODES

GENITALIA

PERINEUM	CYSTOCELE
VULVA	RECTOCELE
VAGINAL VAULT	PROLAPSE
CERVIX	
FUNDUS	
ADNEXAE	

MALE

RECTAL

SPECIAL EXAMINATION

IMPRESSION

TREATMENT

LABORATORY

	Urine		Blood
	COLOR		HBG
	SP GR		RBC
	ALB		WBC
	SUGAR		C P
	MICRO		SED

Figure 2-1B	MEDICAL RECORD

NAME	AGE	SEX	S M D W
ADDRESS	PHONE		DATE
Sponsor	address		
OCCUPATION	REF BY		ACKN

CHIEF COMPLAINT

PRESENT ILLNESS

FAMILY HISTORY	*URINARY TRACT*
MOTHER FATHER	NOCTURIA FREQUENCY
BROTHERS	PAIN BURNING
SISTERS	BLEEDING INFECTION
TB DIAB MALIG	INCONTINENCE
HT DIS NEPH EPILIP	GENITAL TRACT
PSYCH	AGE AT MENST TYPE PERIOD
PAST HISTORY – GENERAL HEALTH	INTERMEN BLEEDING
	AMENORRHEA DYSMENORRHEA
CHILDHOOD DISEASES	VAG DISCH IRRITATION
SC FEV RHEUM FEV ALLERGY	PAINFUL PERIOD
OTHER	L M P
USUAL WEIGHT	CHILDREN L D SB
ACCIDENTS	MARRIED YRS. YOUNGEST CHILD

HABITS COFFEE TOBACCO ALCOHOL	NEURO-MUSCULAR
REVIEW OF SYSTEMS	STRENGTH NERVOUSNESS
E E N T – EYES	SLEEP WORRY
EARS	MUSCULAR PAIN
NOSE	JOINT PAIN
THROAT	ABNORMAL SENSATIONS
NECK	DEFORMITIES
BREASTS	
HEART—LUNGS	**OPERATIONS**
PAIN COUGH	
BLEEDING DYSPNEA	
IRREG EDEMA	
GASTRO-INTESTINAL	**TREATMENTS**
APPETITE DIET	
INDIGESTION PAIN	
NAUSEA VOMITING	
JAUNDICE BLEEDING	**COMMENT**
BOWEL HABITS	
HEMORRHOIDS	
PAIN WITH STOOL ITCHING	
OTHER	

Continued, Figure 2-1B | **PHYSICAL EXAMINATION**

WT	HT	TEMP	BLOOD PRESSURE	PULSE	RESP

GENERAL APPEARANCE

SKIN—SCALP

BLOOD VESSELS

EYES	EARS	NOSE

MOUTH—TEETH

THROAT

NECK

BREASTS

HEART

LUNGS

RIBS

SPINE

ABDOMEN

HERNIA

EXTREMITIES

REFLEXES

LYMPH NODES

GENITALIA

PERINEUM	CYSTOCELE
VULVA	RECTOCELE
VAGINAL VAULT	PROLAPSE
CERVIX	
FUNDUS	
ADNEXAE	

MALE

RECTAL

SPECIAL EXAMINATION

IMPRESSION

TREATMENT

LABORATORY

	URINE	BLOOD
	COLOR	HBG
	SP GR	RBC
	ALB	WBC
	SUGAR	C P
	MICRO	SED

Figure 2-1C   **MEDICAL RECORD**

NAME		AGE	SEX	S M D W
ADDRESS		PHONE		DATE
Sponsor		address		
OCCUPATION		REF BY		ACKN

CHIEF COMPLAINT

PRESENT ILLNESS

FAMILY HISTORY			*URINARY TRACT*	
MOTHER	FATHER		NOCTURIA	FREQUENCY
BROTHERS			PAIN	BURNING
SISTERS			BLEEDING	INFECTION
TB	DIAB	MALIG	INCONTINENCE	
HT DIS	NEPH	EPILIP	GENITAL TRACT	
PSYCH			AGE AT MENST	TYPE PERIOD

PAST HISTORY — GENERAL HEALTH

INTERMEN BLEEDING

AMENORRHEA   DYSMENORRHEA

CHILDHOOD DISEASES			VAG DISCH	IRRITATION
SC FEV	RHEUM FEV	ALLERGY	PAINFUL PERIOD	
OTHER			L M P	
USUAL WEIGHT			CHILDREN L D SB	

ACCIDENTS

MARRIED YRS.   YOUNGEST CHILD

HABITS   COFFEE   TOBACCO   ALCOHOL   NEURO-MUSCULAR

REVIEW OF SYSTEMS		STRENGTH	NERVOUSNESS
E E N T — EYES		SLEEP	WORRY
EARS		MUSCULAR PAIN	
NOSE		JOINT PAIN	
THROAT		ABNORMAL SENSATIONS	
NECK		DEFORMITIES	
BREASTS			

HEART—LUNGS		**OPERATIONS**
PAIN	COUGH	
BLEEDING	DYSPNEA	
IRREG	EDEMA	

GASTRO-INTESTINAL		**TREATMENTS**
APPETITE	DIET	
INDIGESTION	PAIN	
NAUSEA	VOMITING	
JAUNDICE	BLEEDING	**COMMENT**
BOWEL HABITS		
HEMORRHOIDS		
PAIN WITH STOOL ITCHING		
OTHER		

WT	HT	TEMP	BLOOD PRESSURE	PULSE	RESP
GENERAL APPEARANCE					
SKIN—SCALP					
BLOOD VESSELS					
EYES		EARS		NOSE	
MOUTH—TEETH					
THROAT					
NECK					
BREASTS					
HEART					
LUNGS					
RIBS					
SPINE					
ABDOMEN					
HERNIA					
EXTREMITIES					
REFLEXES					
LYMPH NODES					
GENITALIA					
PERINEUM		CYSTOCELE			
VULVA		RECTOCELE			
VAGINAL VAULT		PROLAPSE			
CERVIX					
FUNDUS					
ADNEXAE					
MALE					
RECTAL					

SPECIAL EXAMINATION

IMPRESSION

TREATMENT

LABORATORY

	URINE	BLOOD
	COLOR	HBG
	SP GR	RBC
	ALB	WBC
	SUGAR	C P
	MICRO	SED

Discussion Topics

1. Sleep patterns are often indicators of underlying medical problems. However, patients quite often do not rate this as significant enough to even mention during a routine examination. Discuss how you can encourage patients to elaborate upon their sleep habits. Points mentioned such as irritability, memory loss, episodes of falling asleep uncontrollably, and boredom are examples of important messages indicating sleep problems. Discuss sleep patterns of your classmates or family members to become more familiar with wide variances among populations. Include interviews with family members in different age groups for comparison.

2. Tobacco, drugs, and alcohol are substances that are potentially hazardous to health, including the health of a fetus. Read the following excerpt from a health history and discuss its implications to the patient's overall health:

> This 28-year-old male has smoked cigarettes for the past 10 years. Until one year ago he smoked one pack of cigarettes a day but cut back to six or seven cigarettes per day, mostly following meals or when relaxing after work.
>
> He denies using sedatives, barbiturates, narcotics, amphetamines, or laxatives, stating "I don't like pills." He drinks beer and wine but mostly on weekends when relaxing with friends.

Review and Rationale

Answer the following questions in the space provided.

1. Why is it important to provide a quiet, private environment while taking the patient's history?

____

____

____

2. Why should the medical assistant be present during the physical examination of a female patient when the physician is male?

____

____

____

3. Why would the physician require the patient to be placed in a particular position?

____

____

____

4. Why are drapes and gowns used?

____

____

____

5. Why is it important to be sure the patient is well supported with pillows or a binder while in a particular position?

____

____

____

6. Why is a drape wrapped around the legs and placed under the heels of the feet when the patient is in lithotomy position?

____

____

____

7. Why is it important to place the drape neatly over the patient's abdomen for patients placed in the dorsal-recumbent position?

____

____

____

8. Why is the Sims' or left lateral position frequently used for rectal or vaginal exams on older women?

____

____

____

9. Why should you encourage the patient to give specific information about their medical history?

____

____

____

10. Why is it important to listen carefully to the patient and pay attention to his voice?

____

____

____

Performance Test

In a skills laboratory, a simulation of a job-like environment, the medical assistant student is to demonstrate knowledge and skill in performing the following procedures without reference to source materials. Time limits for the performance of each procedure are to be assigned by the instructor.

Positioning and Draping

Demonstrate proficiency in positioning and draping patients in the following:
1. lithotomy
2. dorsal-recumbent
3. knee-chest
4. Sims'
5. supine
6. prone
7. Fowler's position

You are expected to perform the above activities with 100% accuracy 90% of the time (9 out of 10 times).

Performance Checklist

DIRECTIONS: The following checklist will be used to evaluate your performance of each procedure.

Checklist 2-1: Lithotomy Position

Checklist	S or NA	U	NO	Comment
1. Wash hands.				
2. Explain nature of the examination to the patient.				
3. Prepare room and examining table with paper liner or sheet covering the table.				
4. Request that patient lie on his/her back with legs separated and knees flexed.				
5. Drape patient using diamond technique.				
6. Support feet in stirrups protecting feet with drape.				
7. Provide for the care and comfort of the patient.				
8. Clean the patient as needed and remove soiled linen immediately.				
9. Wash your hands.				
10. Allow patient to rest in supine position for a few minutes before getting up.				

*S or NA = satisfactory or not applicable; U = unsatisfactory; NO = not observed

Checklist 2-2: Dorsal-Recumbent Position

Checklist	S or NA	U	NO	Comment
1. Wash hands.				
2. Explain nature of the examination to the patient.				
3. Prepare room and examining table with paper liner or sheet covering the table, and a small towel under the buttocks area.				
4. Place soles of the feet flat on the table.				
5. Buttocks must be brought to the edge of the examining table.				
6. Drape patient using diamond technique.				
7. Place small towel under the buttocks.				
8. Provide for the care and comfort of the patient.				
9. Clean the patient as needed and remove soiled linen immediately.				
10. Allow patient to rest in supine position for a few minutes before getting up.				

*S or NA = satisfactory or not applicable; U = unsatisfactory; NO = not observed

Checklist 2-3: Knee-Chest Position

Checklist	S or NA	U	NO	Comment
1. Wash hands.				
2. Explain nature of the examination to the patient.				
3. Prepare room and examining table with paper liner or sheet covering the table.				
4. Ask patient to kneel on the table, keeping the buttocks elevated and the back straight.				
5. Place a small pillow under the chest for comfort and support.				
6. Turn the head to one side, and flex the arms at the elbow.				
7. Elbows extend over each side of the exam table.				
8. Place hands under or near the side of the head.				
9. Place the drape sheet as a diamond over the body.				
10. Place smaller sheet over the legs.				
11. When exam begins, pull back the drape sheet and fold it over the top of the buttocks.				
12. Provide for the care and comfort of the patient.				
13. Clean the patient as needed and remove soiled linen immediately.				
14. Wash your hands.				
15. Allow patient to rest in supine position for a few minutes before getting up.				

*S or NA = satisfactory or not applicable; U = unsatisfactory; NO = not observed

Checklist 2-4: Sims' Position (Figure 2-2)

Checklist	S or NA	U	NO	Comment
1. Wash hands.				
2. Explain nature of the examination to the patient.				
3. Prepare room and examining table with paper liner or sheet covering the table.				
4. Instruct patient to lie down on the table and then roll over onto the left side and chest.				
5. Position patient's buttocks near the edge of the side of the exam table.				
6. Left leg is slightly flexed and the right leg is sharply flexed.				
7. Place the left arm behind the patient so that the body is leaning slightly forward.				
8. Position the right arm in front of the body for comfort and support.				
9. Place a small towel under the right arm and knee. Cover the patient with a drape sheet.				
10. As the examination begins, fold back the drape corner so that only the anal and reproductive organ areas are exposed.				
11. Provide for the care and comfort of the patient.				
12. Clean the patient as needed and remove soiled linen immediately.				
13. Wash your hands.				
14. Allow patient to rest in supine position for a few minutes before getting up.				

*S or NA = satisfactory or not applicable; U = unsatisfactory; NO = not observed

Figure 2-2 Illustrates a patient supported with pillows in Sims' position. (From Sorrentino: Mosby's Textbook for Nursing Assistants 3E, St. Louis, 1992, Mosby)

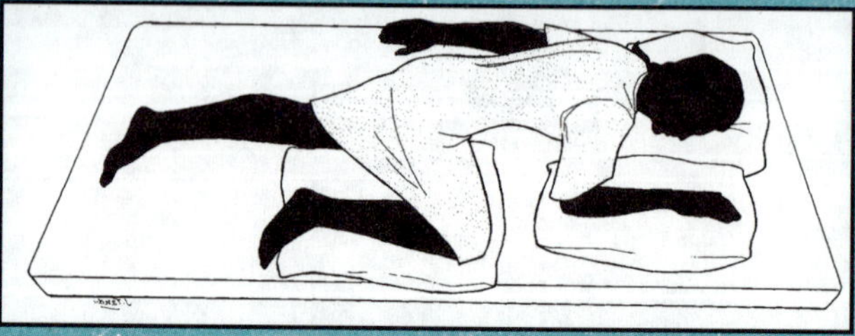

Checklist 2-5: Supine Position (Figure 2-3B)

Checklist	S or NA	U	NO	Comment
1. Wash hands.				
2. Explain nature of the examination to the patient.				
3. Prepare room and examining table with paper liner or sheet covering the table.				
4. Instruct patient to lie flat on his back, with arms placed at his sides and his head elevated on a small pillow.				
5. Provide for the care and comfort of the patient.				
6. Clean the patient as needed and remove soiled linen immediately.				
7. Wash your hands.				
8. Allow patient to rest in supine position for a few minutes before getting up.				

*S or NA = satisfactory or not applicable; U = unsatisfactory; NO = not observed

Figure 2-3

(From Sorrention: Mosby's Textbook for Nursing Assistants 3E, St. Louis, 1992, Mosby)

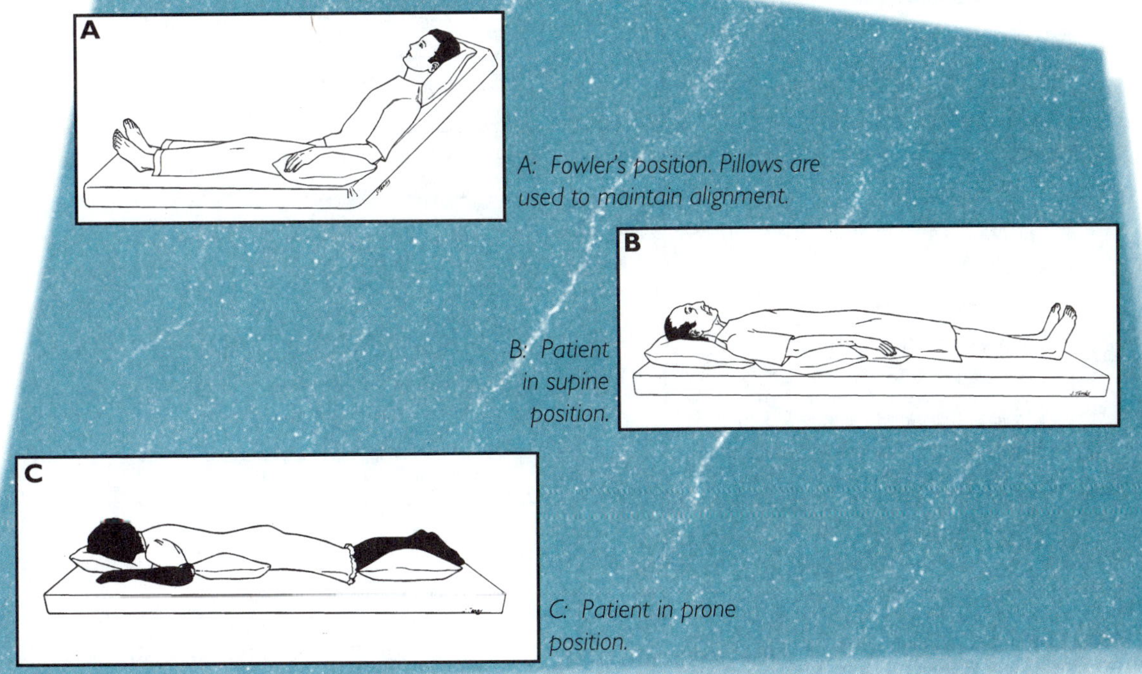

A: Fowler's position. Pillows are used to maintain alignment.

B: Patient in supine position.

C: Patient in prone position.

Checklist 2-6: Prone Position (See Figure 2-3C)

Checklist	S or NA	U	NO	Comment
1. Wash hands.				
2. Explain nature of the examination to the patient.				
3. Prepare room and examining table with paper liner or sheet covering the table.				
4. Instruct the patient to lie flat on his abdomen, arms flexed under the head and head turned to one side.				
5. Provide for the care and comfort of the patient.				
6. Clean the patient as needed and remove soiled linen immediately.				
7. Wash your hands.				
8. Allow patient to rest in supine position for a few minutes before getting up.				

*S or NA = satisfactory or not applicable; U = unsatisfactory; NO = not observed

Checklist 2-7: Fowler's Position (See Figure 2-3A)

Checklist	S or NA	U	NO	Comment
1. Wash hands.				
2. Explain nature of the examination to the patient.				
3. Prepare room and examining table with paper liner or sheet covering the table.				
4. Instruct patient to sit up on the side of the examining table.				
5. Provide for the care and comfort of the patient.				
6. Clean the patient as needed and remove soiled linen immediately.				
7. Wash your hands.				
8. Allow patient to rest in supine position for a few minutes before getting up.				

*S or NA = satisfactory or not applicable; U = unsatisfactory; NO = not observed

Multiple Choice

From the options listed under each question or statement, select the correct answer or answers. Write the corresponding letter or letters in the answer space.

1. The history is a series of questions and answers about the patient's: ________
   a. chief complaint
   b. past, present and family illnesses
   c. personal history
   d. all of the above

2. A general physical exam may require which of the following: ________
   a. tape measure, tuning forks, ophthalmoscope, and otoscope
   b. laryngeal mirror, neurological pin wheel, percussion hammer, alcohol swabs, and cotton balls
   c. stethoscope, thermometer, tongue blade, blood pressure cuff, specimen bottle, and waste container
   d. any of the above

3. The position chosen for the type of examination depends on all except: ________
   a. examination or procedure to be performed
   b. patient's age and sex
   c. patient's preference
   d. physical and emotional condition.

4. Drapes and a gown are used to: ________
   a. protect the patient's privacy
   b. provide comfort
   c. avoid chilling
   d. all of the above

5. Proper draping allows: ________
   a. only the examined part of the body to be exposed
   b. sterile field
   c. comfort for the patient
   d. none of the above

6. The position where the feet are supported in stirrups is called: ________
   a. Sims'
   b. lithotomy
   c. left lateral
   d. Fowler's

7. For vaginal, prostatic, or rectal examination which of the following positions may be used? ________

    a. prone

    b. supine

    c. knee-chest

    d. dorsal recumbent

8. Which position is chosen for rectal exams on older women who are unable to maintain the lithotomy position? ________

    a. Sims'

    b. Trendelenburg

    c. knee-chest

    d. supine

9. The position in which the patient lies flat on his back with arms placed at his sides and head elevated on a small pillow is called: ________

    a. Fowler's

    b. supine

    c. prone

    d. lithotomy

10. While the patient is waiting for the physician to perform the physical examination, the medical assistant may wish to: ________

    a. sterilize instruments

    b. clean up room from previous patient

    c. explain some of the exam techniques the physician will use

    d. begin the exam

True or False

Determine whether each of the following statements is true or false. Check the box marked T or F at the left of the statement.

T   F

☐ ☐   1. Ask the patient about his/her symptoms with questions which answer "what," "where," and "when."

☐ ☐   2. If a patient confides in you with information, you must adhere to patient confidentiality and not say anything to the physician.

☐ ☐   3. The physical examination always involves only the area the patient's chief complaint covers.

☐ ☐   4. The type of equipment needed by the physician depends on the specific physical exam procedure.

T F

☐ ☐ 5. A female assistant must remain in the room if the patient is a male and the physician is male.

☐ ☐ 6. In addition to the general physical set up, the proctoscope, vaginal speculum, or uterine forceps may be required.

☐ ☐ 7. Every examination requires a urine specimen.

☐ ☐ 8. Draw the physician's attention to any information on the health history of significance.

☐ ☐ 9. Light sources and electrical equipment should be tested periodically to assure they are in good working order.

☐ ☐ 10. All patients must disrobe completely and put on a gown regardless of the examination performed.

Word Puzzle

Circle the following medical terms related to the physical exam.

ophthalmoscope	forceps	prone	Fowler
lithotomy	stethoscope	laryngeal	
Sims'	examination	proctoscope	
ROS	supine	speculum	

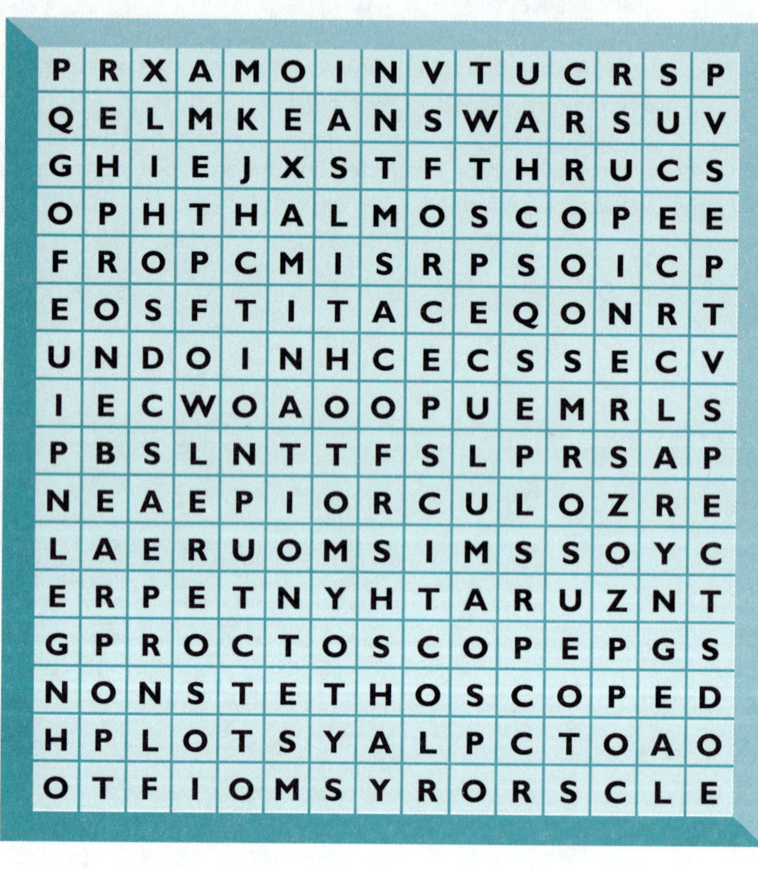

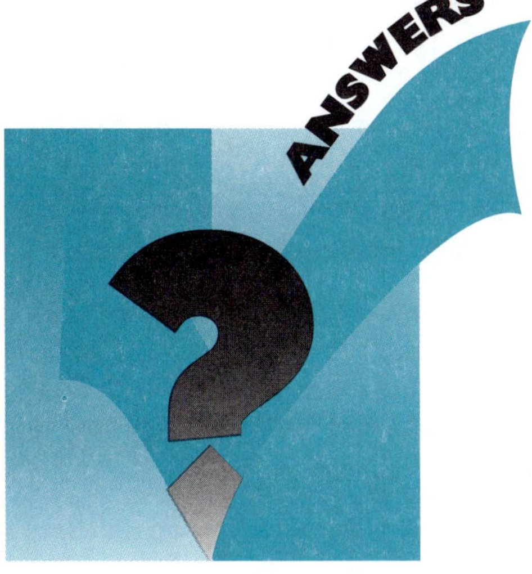

Vocabulary

1. m	4. j	7. f	10. l	13. b
2. h	5. k	8. c	11. n	14. o
3. e	6. a	9. i	12. g	15. d

Student Activities

1–4. Answers may vary.

Discussion Topics

1–2. Answers may vary.

Review and Rationale

1. Successful interviewing begins with your attitude toward the patient. Providing a quiet, private environment while taking a patient's history will encourage discussion of confidential information.

2. Your presence helps an anxious patient to relax, and also protects the physician from unwarranted law suits.

3. Positioning the patient allows the physician better visibility of and accessibility to an area during the examination.

4 Drapes and a gown are for the patient's privacy and modesty while in a given position. They also allow only the examined part of the body to be exposed.

5. Most of the positions are uncomfortable and difficult to maintain for any length of time.

6. Wrap the drape around the legs and heels of the feet for patients placed in lithotomy position to increase comfort.

7. It is important not to allow the drape sheet to fall over the perineum as this would obstruct the physician's view during examination of a patient placed in the dorsal-recumbent position.

8. The Sims' or left lateral position is frequently used for rectal or vaginal exams on older women who are unable to maintain the lithotomy position.

9. Medical problems and personal data including stresses at home or work can help identify factors which may affect the patient's health.

10. If the voice is anxious, upset, or intense with pain, alert the doctor to the patient's comments. He/she may be able to discuss the problem with the patient more thoroughly.

Multiple Choice

1. d	3. c	5. a	7. c	9. b
2. d	4. d	6. b	8. a	10. c

True or False

1. T	3. F	5. F	7. F	9. T
2. F	4. T	6. T	8. T	10. F

Word Puzzle

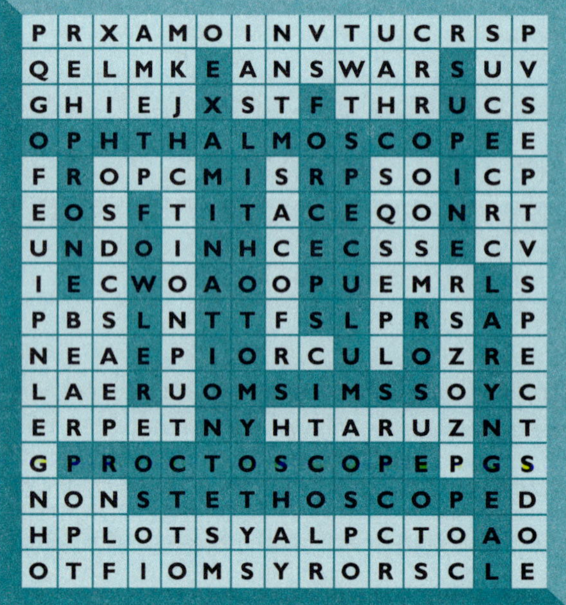

HISTORICAL HIGHLIGHTS

Hippocrates (b.460 B.C.) foreshadowed asepsis when he advocated irrigating wounds with wine or boiled water.

Galen (A.D. 12\31-200), the Greek physician and founder of experimental physiology, boiled instruments used in caring for wounded gladiators.

Girolama Francastoro said in 1546 that contagion was due to the passage of minute bodies, capable of self-multiplication, from the infector to the infected.

Holland-born Leeuwenhoek ground very small lenses out of clear glass to see objects larger than they appeared to the unaided eye.

In 1799 Webster wrote about general epidemiology; Semmelweis (1818–1865) established the etiology of puerperal fever; Pasteur found that heat could halt organisms' growth; Koch was the founder of bacteriology; and Nightingale advocated use of pure air, pure water, efficient drainage, cleanliness, and light for health.

All of those pioneers who followed lead to the sterile techniques and continued progress made today in reducing wound infection and improving the quality of patient care. As a medical assistant, these processes will be part of your daily routine and help keep you and everyone around you safe from infection.

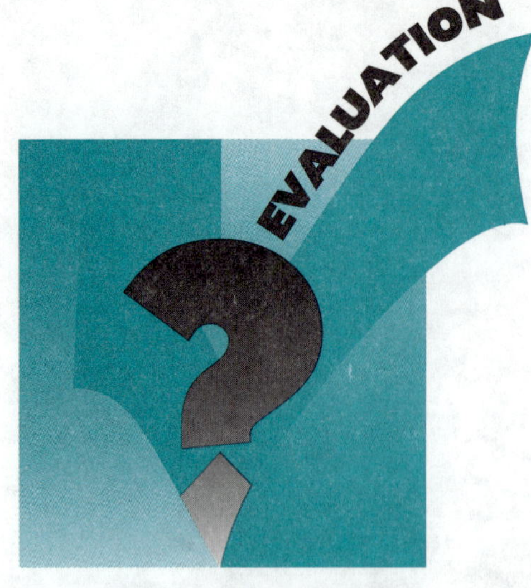

Vocabulary

Write the letter of each term on the line of its matching definition at the right.

a. pathogenic

b. microorganisms

c. bacteria

d. viruses

e. parasites

f. reservoir

g. resistance

h. phagocytes

i. antibodies

j. surgical asepsis

1. _____ protein substances produced in the lymph nodes, spleen and bone marrow, lymphoid tissue

2. _____ the smallest pathogens

3. _____ defense mechanisms

4. _____ microorganisms which cause disease

5. _____ destruction of all microorganisms, pathogenic and nonpathogenic, before entering body

6. _____ "cell eating" cells

7. _____ minute living creatures too small to be seen by the naked eye

8. _____ organisms that live in or on other organisms

9. _____ single-celled organisms which readily multiply outside of living cells

10. _____ site where a pathogenic organism grows and reproduces

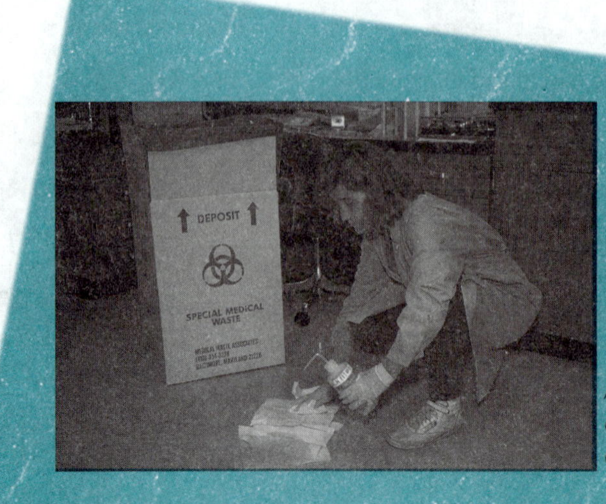

A gloved medical assistant cleans up a body fluid.

Student Activities

Read the following case studies and discuss the *italicized* terminology.

1. Case Study

Description: A 2-year-old child was accompanied by his mother for evaluation of *vesicles* described as *pustular* skin eruptions with yellow crusts.

Etiology: *Streptococcus.* The problem was *exacerbated* by poor hygiene.

Signs and Symptoms: A thick, yellow crust formed over the infected sites—lips and nostrils.

Diagnostic Procedures: Inspection of characteristic *lesions.*

Treatment: Antibiotics and thorough cleansing of the lesions *b.i.d.*

Prognosis: Good

Prevention: Good hygiene and avoidance of infected persons. Child is not to return to day care until lesions are healed.

2. Case Study

Description: This 32-year-old female presented with an acute, chronic infection of the fallopian tubes, ovaries, and adjacent structures diagnosed as *Pelvic Inflammatory Disease (PID).*

Etiology: *Chlamydia*

Signs and Symptoms: Sudden pelvic pain, a purulent and foul-smelling vaginal discharge, fever, and *metrorrhagia,* and rebound pain.

Diagnostic Procedures: A smear of uterine secretions were sent for culture. *Ultrasonography* was ordered to identify any uterine mass.

Treatment: The patient was placed on *antibiotics, analgesics,* and bed rest.

Prognosis: Good

Prevention: None known.

3. Case Study

Description: This 58-year-old patient presented complaining of frequent passage of feces, with an accompanying increase in fluidity and volume.

Etiology: Unknown.

Signs and Symptoms: The diarrhea was accompanied by *flatulence, abdominal distension, anorexia, vomiting,* and *malaise.*

Diagnostic Procedures: Bacterial cultures and microscopic examination of the stools were performed. Stool examination for *occult* blood were positive; therefore, elective *sigmoidoscopy* was performed.

Treatment: Bacterial cultures were positive and patient was placed on the appropriate antibiotic. Patient placed on *BRAT* diet, clear liquids and instructed about the possible complications of *dehydration* and *electrolyte* imbalance.

Prognosis: Good.

Prevention: A high fiber diet or the use of fiber therapy such as Citrucel (methylcellulose) provides a daily source of soluble fiber to the diet.

Discussion Topics

1. Read the following paragraph (From Atkinson "Berry & Kohn's Operating Room Technique," 7/E, St. Louis, 1992, Mosby) and discuss the *italicized* vocabulary and its relationship to infection:

> The quality of life, both physical and psychological, can be drastically altered, sometimes permanently, by infection and the associated "d's": *delayed healing, discomfort, distress, dependency,* and *dollars.* Not infrequently, *disability, deformity,* and *disaster* with ultimate *death* are the result of infection. A mild infection is potentially a severe one.

2. The Infection Control Coordinator at Mercy General Hospital where your physician employer has staff privileges has notified the doctor of an unacceptable infection rate on patients who had procedures performed during the previous month. This program monitors the hospital environment for infections, including all aspects of control activities such as:

   a. investigation of outbreaks of infection above expected levels

   b. identification of origin and etiology of outbreaks by epidemiologic study

   c. tracing factors that contribute to infection problems

    d. consultation in case of clusters of wound infections in infected patients with same procedure, same operating team, or operative problem

Upon review of three patients who had postoperative wound infections following bunionectomy, the doctor asked you to correlate any significant similarities. Using the four activities listed above, discuss how you would conduct the investigation.

3. The office staff has been assigned the responsibility of establishing an infection control policy to include the following:

    a. cleaning, disinfection, and sterilization of equipment,

    b. control of contaminants,

    c. application of aseptic techniques basic to an effective infection control program

        – breaks in asepsis may also result from the intrusion of pests, vermin, insects, noxious substances, chemicals, gases, and infectious body fluids and wastes into the protected areas

        – effective disposal procedures for soiled materials and debris

Discuss the reporting of any breach of policy.

4. Contact local health organizations for current studies being performed on the topic: Antibiotic utilization in the treatment of community-acquired pneumonia.

Review and Rationale

Answer the following questions in the space provided.

1. Why does disease or infection occur when a pathogenic organism invades a human body?

____

____

____

2. How does an infecting organism cause a new infection?

____

____

____

3. Every pathogen gaining entry into the body does not cause disease or infection. What is

the explanation for this?

____

____

____

4. Why must you always use medical and surgical aseptic practices?

____

____

____

5. Why is it important to keep the soap bar from coming into contact with the sink or soap dish while using it?

____

____

____

6. Why is it suggested you turn the faucet off with a paper towel?

____

____

____

7. Why should you consider any exposure to blood or body fluids as potentially dangerous?

____

____

____

8. Why should you use Universal Precautions?

____

____

____

9. Why should you wear gloves when you have a cut or sore on your hand?

____

____

____

10. Why should you wear a mask when caring for a patient whose cough has not been diagnosed?

____

____

____

11. Why should you take great caution when using or disposing of needles?

____

____

____

12. Why should you never leave any needle or sharp instrument on the counter top, on examination tables, or on disposable procedure trays?

____

____

____

13. Why should paper towels used to clean up spills of blood and body fluids be placed in an infectious waste container?

____

____

____

14. Why is it incorrect to use undiluted bleach for cleaning purposes?

____

____

____

15. Why does following Universal Precautions help to promote a clean, safe environment for you, your patients, and your fellow healthcare workers?

____

____

____

Performance Test

In a skills laboratory, a simulation of a job-like environment, the medical assistant student must demonstrate knowledge and skill in performing the following procedure without reference to source materials. For this activity the student will need gloves, gowns, goggles and masks, sink with water and soap. Time limits for the performance of the procedure are to be assigned by the instructor.

1. Handwashing Technique

You are expected to perform these activities with 100% accuracy 90% of the time (9 out of 10 times).

Performance Checklist

DIRECTIONS: The following checklist will be used to evaluate your performance of each procedure.

Checklist 3-1: Proper Handwashing Technique

Checklist	S or NA	U	NO	Comment
1. Remove your watch and place it in your pocket, or if it has an elastic band, it may be moved higher up your arm.				
2. Turn on the water and adjust the water to a lukewarm setting.				
3. Wet your hands and apply enough soap to develop a good lather. Do not contaminate the soap.				
4. Vigorously wash your palms, sides and backs of hands using a rubbing motion.				
5. Wash between your fingers and around your knuckles. (Figure 3-1)				
6. Clean under your nails with an orangewood stick or nail brush.				
7. Rinse nails well under running water without letting water run onto hands.				
8. Turn off the water with a paper towel.				
9. Use clean paper towel to thoroughly dry your hands, wrist and forearms.				

*S or NA = satisfactory or not applicable; U = unsatisfactory; NO = not observed

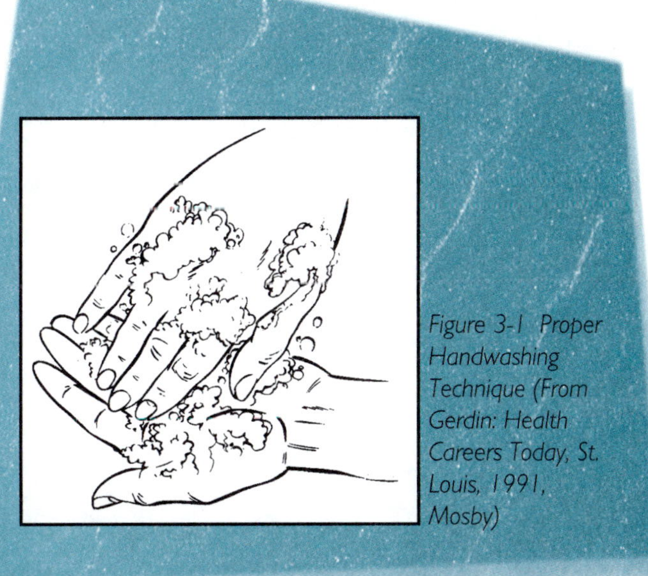

Figure 3-1 Proper Handwashing Technique (From Gerdin: Health Careers Today, St. Louis, 1991, Mosby)

Multiple Choice

From the options listed under each question or statement, select the correct answer or answers. Write the corresponding letter or letters in the answer space.

1. Disease or infection occurs when: _________
   a. body resistance is low
   b. the body is unable to fight
   c. a pathogenic organism invades a human body
   d. none of the above

2. Bacteria are defined as: _________
   a. minute living creatures
   b. viruses and parasites
   c. the smallest pathogens
   d. single-celled organisms which can readily multiply outside of living cells

3. Parasites are organisms that live: _________
   a. in nose, mouth, and laryngeal fossae
   b. in or on other organisms
   c. in warm, moist environs
   d. in reservoirs

4. What is the best method for infection control? _________
   a. prevent the spread of disease-producing microorganisms
   b. administer an antibiotic
   c. educate patients
   d. eliminate beneficial organisms

5. The most common pathogenic organisms which cause diseases are: _________
   a. viruses, bacteria, and parasites
   b. bacteria, flu, and fungi
   c. living cells
   d. single-celled organisms

6. Name physical barriers to invading microorganisms: _________
   a. cilia-lined respiratory tract
   b. nasal mucosa and hair lining the nostrils
   c. skin
   d. all of the above

7. Infection begins when: _______
   a. the sterile field is broached
   b. organisms readily multiply
   c. a high concentration of pathogenic organisms invade the body
   d. a patient's immune system falters

8. Chemical barriers of the skin such as an acidic pH and sweat: _______
   a. inhibit pathogen development
   b. encourage reproduction of cells
   c. inhibit bacterial infection
   d. none of the above

9. Name a common pus-producing organism found in pimples, boils, and suture abscesses.: _______
   a. bacteria
   b. staphylococci
   c. viruses
   d. AIDS

True or False

Determine whether each of the following statements is true or false. Check the box marked T or F at the left of the statement.

T F

☐ ☐ 1. All microorganisms are harmful to humans.

☐ ☐ 2. Disease-causing microorganisms cannot be spread from inanimate objects to humans.

☐ ☐ 3. The best control of infections is treatment with antibiotics.

☐ ☐ 4. Infection begins when a high concentration of pathogenic organisms invade the body.

☐ ☐ 5. Parasites are among the most common pathogenic organisms.

☐ ☐ 6. Staphylococci bacteria are common pus-producing organisms.

☐ ☐ 7. Reservoirs are only found in human beings and animals.

☐ ☐ 8. A new infection is caused only when it finds a way into a new, susceptible host.

T F

☐ ☐   9. An infecting organism can cross the placenta.

☐ ☐   10. Resistance is the body's defense mechanism.

Word Puzzle

Fill in each line with a word related to Infection Control from the video or workbook that fits the definitions below. When the puzzle is completed, the highlighted vertical column will answer the question: "What technique destroys all microorganisms, pathogenic, and nonpathogenic before they enter the body?"

_______________ 1. test using inaudible sounds with frequencies greater than 20,000 cycles per second to produce an image of an organ or tissue

_______________ 2. excessive gas in the stomach and intestines

_______________ 3. a minute organism not visible with ordinary light microscopy

_______________ 4. ejecting material from the stomach through the mouth

_______________ 5. an organism capable of producing a disease

_______________ 6. pertaining to a basin-like structure

_______________ 7. a microorganism that causes a wide variety of diseases in man and animals

_______________ 8. a single-celled organism which readily multiplies outside of living cells

_______________ 9. drugs used to treat infections

_______________ 10. drugs that relieve pain

_______________ 11. protein substances produced in the lymph nodes, spleen and bone marrow, lymphoid tissue

_______________ 12. defense mechanisms

_______________ 13. permanent cessation of all vital functions

_______________ 14. cells that eat cells

_______________ 15. material spread on a surface for examination and diagnosis

_______________ 16. organism that lives in or on other organisms

_______________ 17. a pathologic condition of the body presenting clinical signs and symptoms

Video 3: Infection Control

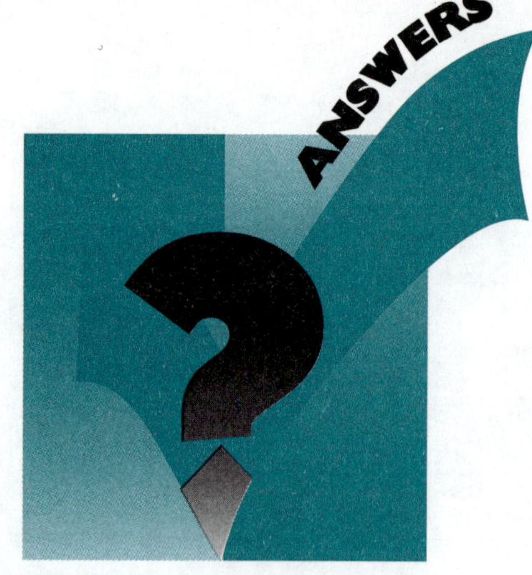

Vocabulary

1. i	3. g	5. j	7. b	9. c
2. d	4. a	6. h	8. e	10. f

Student Activities

1. Case Study Definitions:
   a. *vesicles* - a small sac containing fluid
   b. *pustular* - pertaining to a small elevation of skin filled with lymph or pus
   c. *streptococcus* - a twisted, berry shaped bacteria
   d. *exacerbated* - an increase in the seriousness of a disease as marked by greater intensity in the symptoms
   e. *lesions* - a circumscribed area of pathologically altered tissue
   f. *b.i.d.* - administered two times a day

2. Case Study Definitions:
   a. *Pelvic Inflammatory Disease (PID)* - includes infection of the cervix, uterus, and ovaries
   b. *Chlamydia* - a microorganism that causes a wide variety of diseases in man and animals
   c. *metrorrhagia* - bleeding from the uterus other than during the menstrual period
   d. *ultrasonography* - a test using inaudible sounds with frequencies greater than 20,000 cycles per second to produce an image of an organ or tissue
   e. *antibiotics* - an antimicrobial agent used to treat infections
   f. *analgesics* - drugs that relieve pain

3. Case Study Definitions:
   a. *flatulence* - excessive gas in the stomach and intestines
   b. *abdominal distention* - state of abdomen being stretched or inflated
   c. *anorexia* - loss of appetite

d. *vomiting* - or ejecting material from the stomach through the mouth

e. *malaise* - discomfort, uneasiness, or indisposition, often indicative of infection

f. *occult* - hidden

g. *sigmoidoscopy* - examination of the S-shaped portion of the lower colon (sigmoid) with an instrument called a sigmoidoscope

h. *BRAT* - special diet consisting of bananas, rice, applesauce, and toast

i. *dehydration* - removal of water

j. *electrolyte* - ionized salts in blood, tissue fluids and cells of the body

Discussion Topics

1–4. Answers may vary.

Review and Rationale

1. Disease or infection occurs when a pathogenic organism invades a human body whose resistance is so low, it is unable to fight off the invading organism.

2. An infecting organism that has left its reservoir causes a new infection only if it finds a way into a new, susceptible host.

3. Even though a pathogen gains entry to the body, disease or infection may not develop because the body normally has defense mechanisms, called resistance, to protect itself from pathogenic invasion.

4. In order to control and prevent the spread of disease, you must always use medical and surgical aseptic practices.

5. When using bar soap, keep it from getting contaminated.

6. When turning off the water, consider that the faucet is also a contaminated vehicle.

7. You risk exposure to a number of infectious diseases when you come in contact with blood or body fluids.

8. You must know how to protect yourself, your patients, and other healthcare workers by using Universal Precautions.

9. Wearing gloves when you have a cut or sore on your hand will protect both you and the patient from pathogenic invasion.

10. He or she may have tuberculosis. Using protective garments will help to protect you and your patient.

11. Used needles can spread disease and their proper disposal protects you, the physician,

and the janitorial staff from possible contact with blood through unexpected needle sticks.

12. Discard needles immediately in a sharps container that is designed to protect janitorial staff from cutting or sticking themselves while cleaning.

13. Placing contaminated towels in a regular waste container could spread disease to others.

14. In order to protect yourself from noxious fumes, do not use undiluted bleach for cleaning purposes.

15. Following the precautions breaks the infectious cycle which helps promote a clean, safe environment for you, your patients, and your fellow healthcare workers.

Multiple Choice

1. c	3. b	5. a	7. c	9. b
2. d	4. a	6. d.	8. c	

True or False

1. F	3. F	5. T	7. F	9. T
2. F	4. T	6. T	8. T	10. T

Word Puzzle

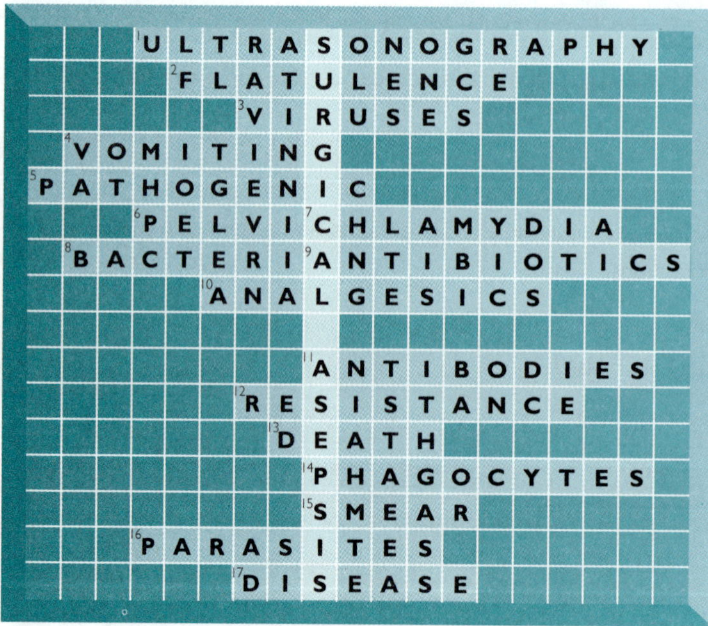

HISTORICAL HIGHLIGHTS

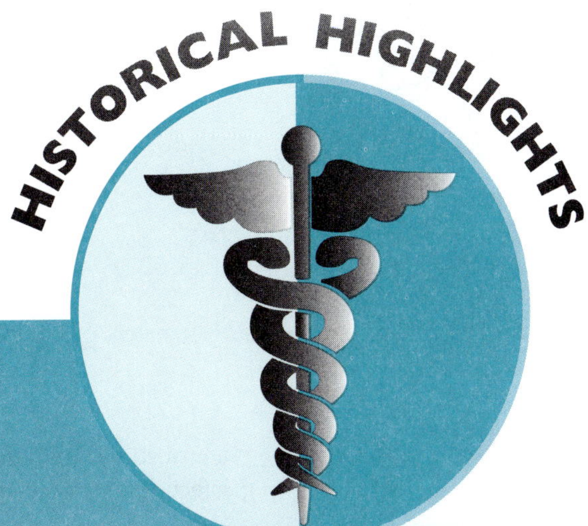

Sterilization by boiling was introduced in the 1880s. Everything used during an operation, including linens, dressings, and gowns was boiled. By 1876 heat-resistant bacteria were demonstrated and by 1886, Ernst von Bergmann and his associates introduced the steam sterilizer. This was soon discovered to be inadequate for sterilization since steam must be under pressure to raise the temperature sufficiently to kill heat-resistant microorganisms. Pressure steam sterilizers were developed to kill resistant spores. This was followed by vacuum-type pressure sterilizers and hot air sterilizers.

Used as a fumigant for insects in the early 20th century, ethylene oxide was recognized as an antibacterial agent around 1929. Sterilization by irradiation developed thereafter.

Coincidental with the development of sterilization, the refinement of operative technique by William Halsted, use of controlled environment, modern operating room attire, and precise housekeeping methods evolved. Over the years sterilization methods were replaced by other sterilization methods, each more effective than its predecessor. Glutaraldehyde, a chemical first introduced in 1963, was approved by the Environmental Protection Agency (FPA) as a sterilant for heat-sensitive instruments.

Active practice of sterile techniques prevents the spread of microorganisms and protects the health and life of your patients and yourself.

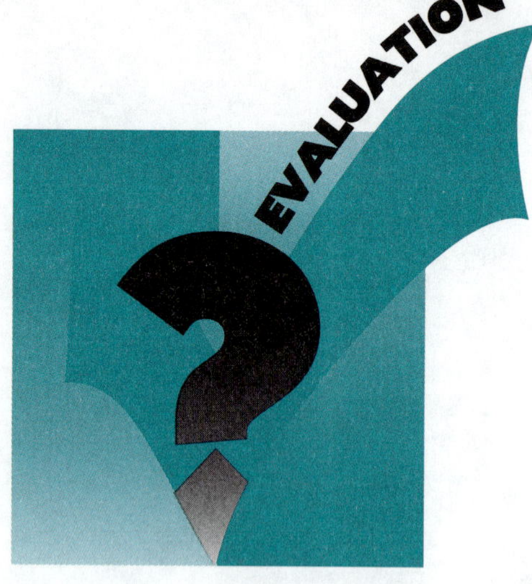

Vocabulary

Write the letter of each term on the line of its matching definition at the right.

a. medical asepsis

b. surgical asepsis

c. sterile technique

d. sanitization

e. disinfection

f. sterilization

g. ultrasonic technique

h. steam sterilization

i. autoclave

j. contamination

k. shelf life

1. _______ a procedure which destroys most, but not all, infectious microorganisms

2. _______ introduction of disease germs or infectious material onto normally sterile objects

3. _______ process of cleansing and scrubbing items with a blood solvent detergent or with chemicals

4. _______ destruction of all pathogenic and nonpathogenic microorganisms before they enter the body

5. _______ sound frequencies above 20,000 cycles per second used to clean medical and surgical instruments

6. _______ another name for surgical asepsis

7. _______ length of time a pack may be considered sterile

8. _______ destruction of organisms after they leave the body

9. _______ most practical means of sterilizing surgical instruments

10. _______ complete destruction of all forms of microscopic life

11. _______ an appliance used to sterilize medical instruments with steam under pressure

Student Activities

1. Contact three medical practices and ask the following questions:

    a. sterilization techniques and methods employed

    b. sterilizing agents used:
       - steam under pressure
       - ethylene oxide gas
       - chemical
       - hot air-dry heat
       - radiation
       - others

    c. types of objects normally sterilized

    d. control measures (for example: spore strips to test steam under pressure)

    e. determination of shelf life and method to inventory sterilized items

2. While performing routine quality assurance procedures for the sterilization of instruments in the doctor's office, the medical assistant noticed water spots left on the instruments. Knowing this can lead to breakdown of the metal, subsequent rusting, and expensive replacement of instruments, what can be done to halt this reaction?

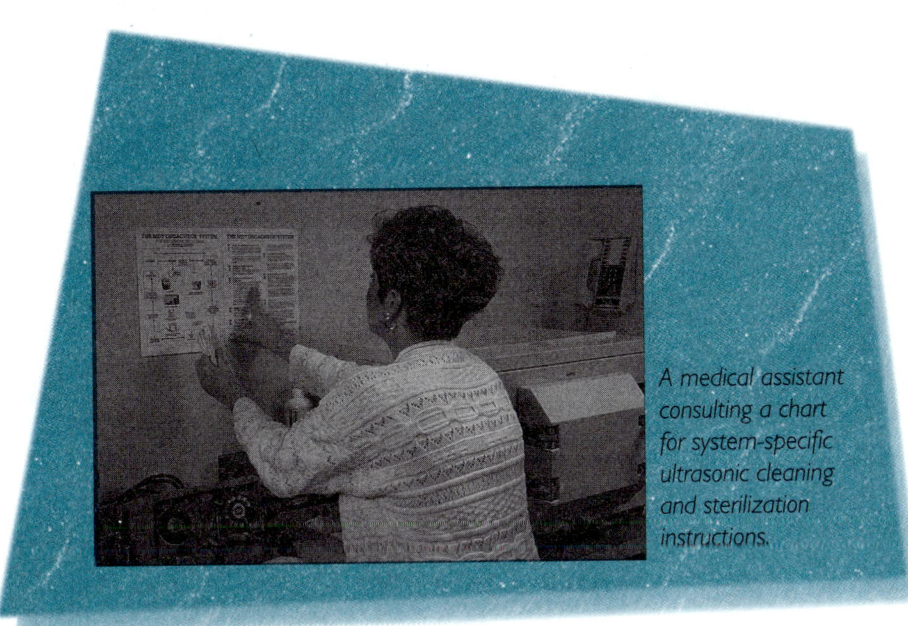

A medical assistant consulting a chart for system-specific ultrasonic cleaning and sterilization instructions.

Discussion Topics

1. The principle of Universal Precautions must be strictly followed when handling instruments with sharp edges contaminated with human blood and fluid products. Discuss the proper steps to follow when applying this principle to the following scenario:

A medical assistant has lacerated her finger with a contaminated knife blade while sanitizing a tray of instruments.

2. When coming into contact with chemicals and agents used to sanitize and disinfect instruments, the medical assistant developed **contact dermatitis** on her hand. Discuss the implications of such an **occupational hazard** and the importance of **OSHA** regulations. What resource information should be available to each worker about the chemicals? What are **MSDS?** Define the *italicized* words.

3. The medical assistant was unloading the autoclave and discovered that the light source for an endoscope had been placed in the pan for sterilization. The scope was now inoperable and the light source had disintegrated. Discuss what steps the medical assistant might institute during the cleaning and sanitizing phase to prevent this costly error.

4. Loud, unusual sounds were coming from the autoclave when the medical assistant entered the room to check what was wrong. At that moment steam spewed out, filling the entire room. The autoclave had malfunctioned and released its steam. What safety precaution should the medical assistant follow to prevent injury?

Review and Rationale

Answer the following questions in the space provided.

1. Why is it important to follow medical and surgical aseptic practices?

____

____

____

2. Why do you wear safety or personal glasses, heavy rubber gloves with long cuffs over disposable gloves, and a plastic apron or fluid resistance gown when sanitizing contaminated items?

____

____

____

3. Why do you use a hand brush or preferably a brush with a handle to scrub items?

____

____

____

4. Why do you roll instruments in a towel?

____

____

____

5. Why is it important to check that all articles are thoroughly clean and in good working condition and alignment?

____

____

____

6. Why should you check that serrations meet evenly; that instruments open and close easily; that all parts are present and intact; and that ratchets close easily and do not spring open?

____

____

____

7. Why do you coat each instrument with a water soluble lubricant such as instrument milk?

____

____

____

8. Why is it unnecessary to hand scrub instruments that will be processed by ultrasonic sanitization?

____

____

____

9. Why must instruments be thoroughly rinsed in cold running water following cleaning in an ultrasonic device?

____

____

____

10. Why do instruments and equipment such as thermometers, percussion hammers, and laryngeal mirrors only need to be disinfected?

____

____

____

11. Why should you follow the manufacturer's recommended directions for using a disin-fectant solution?

____

____

____

12. Why it is important to leave the items in the solution for the required time when dis-infecting?

____

____

____

13. Why is it necessary to disinfect sphygmomanometers, stethoscopes, and ophthalmo-scopes by wiping them with gauze or cloth moistened with a disinfectant?

____

____

____

14. Why is the disinfectant procedure limited in its usefulness?

____

____

____

15. Why must the pack be re-sterilized if the color change standard is not met?

____

____

____

16. Why is it important to note any change in autoclave temperature or pressure, or a less than required steam cycle?

____

____

____

17. Why should items be placed in the autoclave so that the steam can flow between the packs?

____

____

____

18. Why should you exhaust the steam pressure from the chamber before you unload the autoclave?

____

____

____

19. Why should you open the autoclave door only slightly and allow the contents to dry for approximately 15 minutes before removing them?

____

____

____

20. Why can wrapped items placed in sterile plastic dust covers be stored for only six months?

____

____

____

Performance Test

In a skills laboratory, a simulation of a job-like environment, the medical assistant student must demonstrate knowledge and skill in performing the following procedures without reference to source materials. For these activities you will need personal protective equipment, heavy rubber gloves with long cuffs, disposable gloves, fluid resistant apron or gown, and a variety of equipment and instruments required to complete the following skills. Time limits for the performance of each procedure are to be assigned by the instructor.

1. sanitization

2. disinfection

3. sterilization

You are expected to perform these activities with 100% accuracy 90% of the time (9 out of 10 times).

Performance Checklist

DIRECTIONS: The following checklist will be used to evaluate your performance of each procedure.

Checklist 4-1: Sanitization

Checklist	S or NA	U	NO	Comment
1. Don personal protective equipment, including heavy rubber gloves with long cuffs over disposable gloves and a fluid resistant gown or apron.				
2. Rinse items in water containing a blood solvent, low-sudsing detergent, or approved germicide solution.				
3. Clean off all debris, oil, blood, or grease.				
4. Rinse instruments in another sink or pan of fresh water, then scrub each item thoroughly using dishwashing or laundry detergent and a hand brush or preferably a brush with a handle.				
5. Using hot water, thoroughly rinse all detergent from each instrument.				
6. Remove excess moisture from the instruments by rolling them in a towel.				
7. Check that all articles are thoroughly clean and that they are in good working condition and alignment.				
8. Check that all instruments are complete and in good working order.				
9. Coat instrument with instrument milk or water soluble lubricant.				
10. Air dry for 20 minutes.				

*S or NA = satisfactory or not applicable; U = unsatisfactory; NO = not observed

Checklist 4-2: Disinfection Using Disinfectant Solution

Checklist	S or NA	U	NO	Comment
1. Don personal protective equipment, including heavy rubber gloves with long cuffs over disposable gloves and a fluid resistant gown or apron.				
2. Pour the chemical solution into a container with an airtight cover.				
3. Place previously sanitized instruments in a tray, opening all instruments that have handles.				
4. Completely immerse the tray into the solution and close the cover.				
5. Leave items in the solution for the required time.				
6. After correct exposure time has elapsed, with gloved hands, lift tray out of the chemical and rinse items in a pan of sterile distilled water.				
7. Use sterile transfer forceps to remove items from the tray and place them in their specific work area.				

*S or NA = satisfactory or not applicable; U = unsatisfactory; NO = not observed

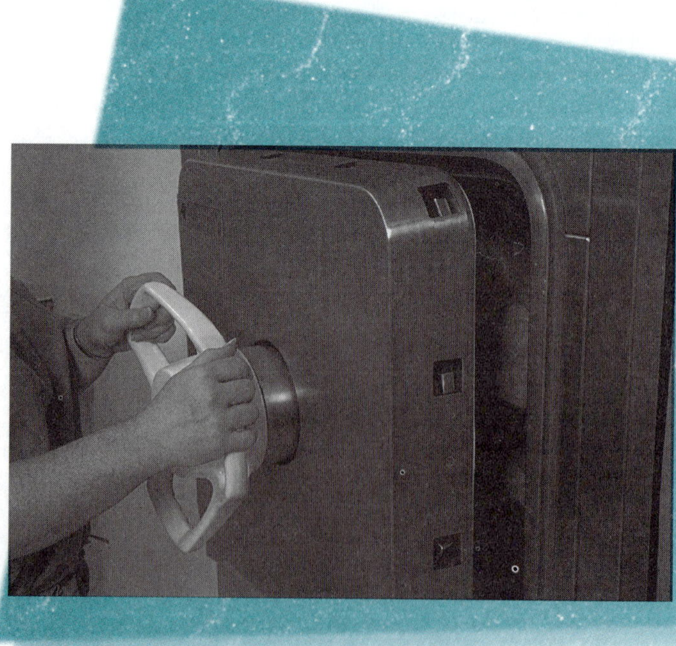

Figure 4-1 When the sterilization cycle is finished, "crack" open the door slightly and allow the contents to dry for 15 minutes before removing them.

Checklist 4-3: Sterilization by Autoclave

Checklist	S or NA	U	NO	Comment
1. Don personal protective equipment, including heavy rubber gloves with long cuffs over disposable gloves and a fluid resistant gown or apron.				
2. Check previously sanitized instruments for good working order and alignment.				
3. Place item on cloth or disposable paper so edges form a diamond pattern.				
4. Place item in the center (hinged items open).				
5. Fold bottom corner up to the item and then double back a small corner.				
6. Fold right side to the item, doubling back a small corner.				
7. Fold left side to the right side and double back that corner.				
8. Pack is folded up from the bottom; top corner is overlapped, and secured with pressure-sensitive tape.				
9. Apply a sterile indicator, following directions for type used.				
10. Date and label contents.				
11. Load autoclave correctly to allow for proper steam flow between packs and penetration.				
12. Demonstrate following manufacturer's recommended procedure for correct operation of autoclave.				
13. Discharge steam from sterilizer according to manufacturer's recommended procedure.				
14. Exhaust steam pressure from the chamber. Observe that pressure has reached zero and temperature is below 212 degrees F.				
15. Open autoclave door slightly; allow contents to dry for 15 minutes before removing them. (See Figure 4-1)				
16. Remove dry, wrapped and unwrapped items that need not remain sterile with clean, dry hands. Check validity of sterile indicator.				
17. Remove unwrapped sterile items with sterile transfer forceps and place items in a sterile environment or sterile storage container.				

*S or NA = satisfactory or not applicable; U = unsatisfactory; NO = not observed

Multiple Choice

From the options listed under each question or statement, select the correct answer or answers. Write the corresponding letter or letters in the answer space.

1. Medical and surgical aseptic practices break the infectious disease cycle so that microorganisms: _______
   a. have an acceptable environment
   b. cannot spread to and invade a susceptible host
   c. are unable to fight off invading organisms
   d. spread directly from person to person

2. Examples of medical aseptic practices are: _______
   a. hand washing
   b. use of gloves when handling highly contaminated articles
   c. cleaning of nondisposable equipment before and after patient use
   d. all of the above

3. The goal of surgical asepsis is to: _______
   a. destroy nonpathogenic microorganisms before they enter the body
   b. destroy organisms after they leave the body
   c. maintain level of infection from spreading
   d. prevent infection or the introduction of microorganisms into the body

4. The primary methods used for inhibiting and destroying microorganism growth are: _______
   a. sanitization, disinfection, and sterilization
   b. disinfection, sanitizing
   c. decontamination, autoclaving, chemical sanitization
   d. radiation and ultrasonic technique

5. Which procedure destroys most, but not all, infectious microorganisms? _______
   a. sanitization
   b. sterilization
   c. disinfection
   d. sanitation

6. If instruments are going to penetrate the skin or mucous membranes, they must be: _______
   a. boiled
   b. irradiated
   c. sterilized
   d. disinfected

7. Items are sanitized through: _______
   a. bulk rinsing in water containing a blood solvent
   b. low-sudsing detergent
   c. an approved germicide solution
   d. all of the above

8. Instruments must be coated with a solution to protect them from corrosion and provide lubrication for the hinges such as: ________
   a. instrument milk
   b. water soluble lubricant
   c. pre-lube solution
   d. all of the above

9. Instruments such as thermometers, percussion hammers, and laryngeal mirrors are examples of items that must be: ________
   a. sterilized
   b. disinfected
   c. autoclaved
   d. none of the above

10. Devices providing assurance that items are sterile as long as wrapper or container is not torn or opened are called: ________
   a. saturation indicator
   b. sterile label
   c. disposable tags
   d. chemical indicators

True or False

Determine whether each of the following statements is true or false. Check the box marked T or F at the left of the statement.

T   F

❏ ❏   1. Clean off all debris, oil, blood or grease prior to sterilization.

❏ ❏   2. It is necessary to sanitize instruments prior to disinfection or wrapping for sterilization.

❏ ❏   3. Instruments cleansed ultrasonically avoid the need for hand scrubbing.

❏ ❏   4. Thermometers and laryngeal mirrors must be sterilized.

❏ ❏   5. Use all chemical full strength for most effective sterilization.

❏ ❏   6. Remove sterilized items from autoclave by hand.

❏ ❏   7. Sphygmomanometers and stethoscopes need only be sanitized.

❏ ❏   8. Boiling water is effective for sterilization.

❏ ❏   9. Steam-under-pressure is accomplished with an appliance called the autoclave.

❏ ❏   10. Disinfection destroys spore-forming bacteria.

Word Puzzle

Circle the following medical terms related to sterilization and disinfection procedures.

sanitization	autoclave	instruments
disinfection	contamination	MSDS
steam	radiation	sterilization
sterile	chemical	asepsis
ultrasonic	ethylene	

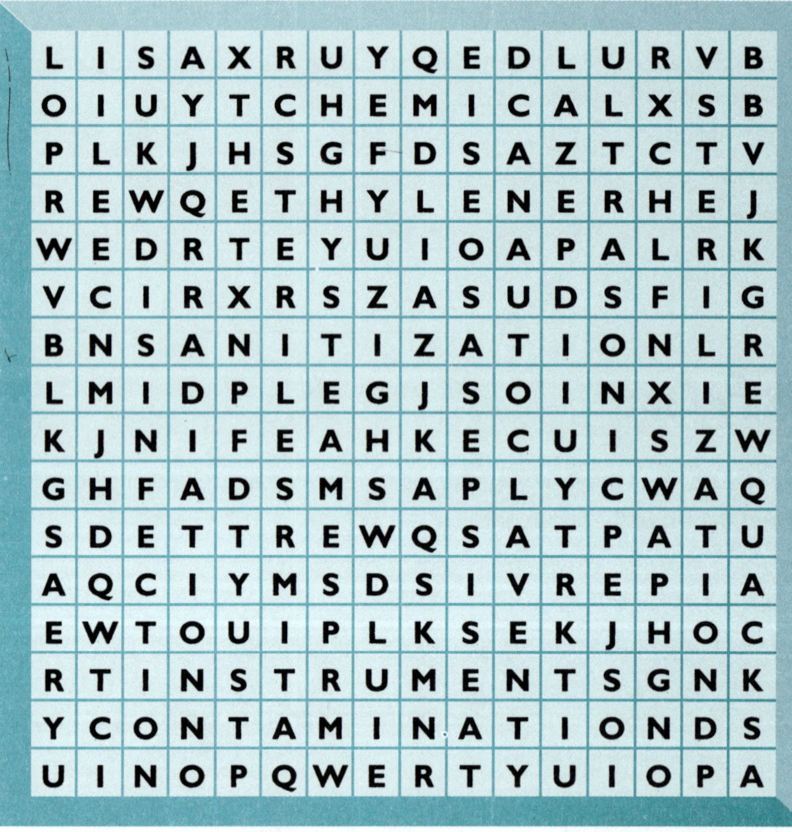

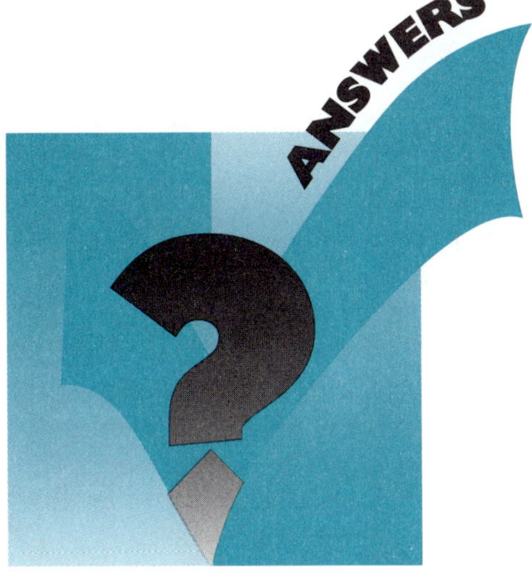

Vocabulary

1. e	3. d	5. g	7. k	9. h	11. i
2. j	4. b	6. c	8. a	10. f	

Student Activities

1. Answers may vary.

2. Answers may vary.

   Suggestions:

   a. Contact vendors of sterilization equipment and supplies.

   b. Consider the water, chemicals, and equipment used in determining what could be causing the water spots.

Discussion Topics

1. Suggestions about what to do if an exposure occurs:

   a. make area bleed a little

   b. report exposure to employer (should be done immediately and by law must be done within 72 hours of the exposure incident)

   c. provide information concerning circumstances and route of exposure, source patient's name, if known

   d. employer must provide an immediate, confidential medical evaluation

   e. HIV testing of source is done if exposure is certified as significant by a physician:

      Exposed employee is requested to have baseline HIV test. If employee refuses baseline testing, no further followup for HIV testing of source patient is done. If employee consents to HIV testing, informed consent for HIV testing is obtained from source patient. If patient is known to be HIV+, no HIV testing is done on source. If patient refuses and blood is available from before the exposure incident, the test is performed. Patient must agree to disclose results of test to employee and employee must be counseled regarding confidentiality of results.

f. HBV testing of source. If source is known to be HBV+, then source is not tested. If HBV status of patient is unknown, source is requested to have blood tested for HBV. If positive, exposed patient starts HB vaccine and receives immunoglobulin. If exposed employee has received HBV vaccine, employee antibody level is tested, if low or absent, booster is given

g. exposed employee must be counseled about any illness that may develop as a result of this exposure

h. the healthcare professional that performs the medical evaluation must provide the employee and employer a written opinion regarding the exposure within 15 days of the evaluation. Report must include whether HBV vaccination was indicated and if employee received it; confirmation that employee has been informed of the results of the evaluation and informed of any medical conditions that may result from their exposure.

2. Answer may vary about implications of such a scenario.

Definitions:

contact dermatitis - inflammation of the skin caused by a primary chemical irritant

occupational hazard - a risk from the work environment

OSHA - Occupational Safety and Health Act/Administration. Government regulations enforced by OSHA include the 1983 "right-to-know" regulations in its standards requiring employees to have access to MSDS.

MSDS - Material Safety Data Sheet. Supplied by each manufacturer for a hazardous chemical in the workplaces, the MSDS must specify:

a. chemical by composition and common names

b. chemical and physical properties

c. known acute and chronic health effects, such as carcinogenic, mutagenic, or allergenic

d. exposure limits

e. protective measures

f. antidote or first-aid measures

3. Answers may vary.

4. The potential for injury exists whenever the autoclave malfunctions. The medical assistant should be knowledgeable of the contents and location of the operations manual and following the manufacturer's suggested recommendations.

Review and Rationale

1. Medical and surgical aseptic practices break the infectious disease cycle so that microorganisms cannot spread to and invade a susceptible host.

2. When sanitizing contaminated items, wear safety or personal glasses, heavy rubber gloves with long cuffs over disposable gloves, and a plastic apron or fluid resistant gown to protect yourself from contact with contaminated items.

3. Use a hand brush or preferably a brush with a handle so that you avoid hand contact with the instrument.

4. Roll instruments in a towel to remove excess moisture.

5. Special attention must be given to scrubbing items with serrated edges where blood or grease may collect and that hot water is used to thoroughly rinse all detergent off each instrument. Any imperfections must be removed during the cleaning process until the item meets quality standards for sterilization.

6. If imperfections are found, remove the item and follow your agency's policy for dealing with broken equipment.

7. Coating each instrument with a water soluble lubricant such as instrument milk, which is a pre-lube solution, protects it from corrosion and provides lubrication for the hinges.

8. Instruments cleansed ultrasonically do not need hand scrubbing, thus avoiding the possibility of transmitting pathogenic microorganisms among patients and medical personnel.

9. Instruments must be thoroughly rinsed in cold, running water to remove residue or ultrasonic solution or soap which might inhibit sterilization or damage the sterilizer.

10. Instruments and equipment such as thermometers, percussion hammers, and laryngeal mirrors come in contact only with the patient's skin or shallow body orifices and may be disinfected.

11. Always follow the manufacturer's recommended directions for using a disinfectant solution, because chemicals may differ in their dilution ratio.

12. Correct exposure time to a disinfectant solution is extremely important to ensure complete disinfection. Disinfection destroys or inhibits disease-producing microorganisms outside the body.

13. Chemical solutions are often toxic and must be thoroughly rinsed from the instruments before they are used on patients.

14. Disinfection procedures can be effective in controlling many forms of microbial life, but may not destroy viruses or spore-forming bacteria. Disinfection procedures must not be substituted for sterilization.

15. Sterilization is assured if the indicator changes color completely, denoting proper sterilization.

16. A change in autoclave temperature or pressure, or a less than required steam cycle, may affect the sterilization process.

17. All items must be placed in the autoclave so that the steam can flow between the

packs and penetrate them. This allows cool air to drain out in a downward direction and then be replaced by steam rather than being trapped inside.

18. Steam under pressure may cause severe injury if the door to the autoclave is opened before or during the exhaust phase.

19. If you open the sterilizer door completely, condensation due to the outside cool air will occur, resulting in wet packs.

20. A six-month recommended period of shelf life is a sterilization standard. After that time, all packs should be reprocessed and re-sterilized before use.

Multiple Choice

1. b	3. d	5. c	7. d	9. b
2. d	4. a	6. c	8. d	10. d

True or False

1. T	3. T	5. F	7. F	9. T
2. T	4. F	6. F	8. F	10. F

Word Puzzle

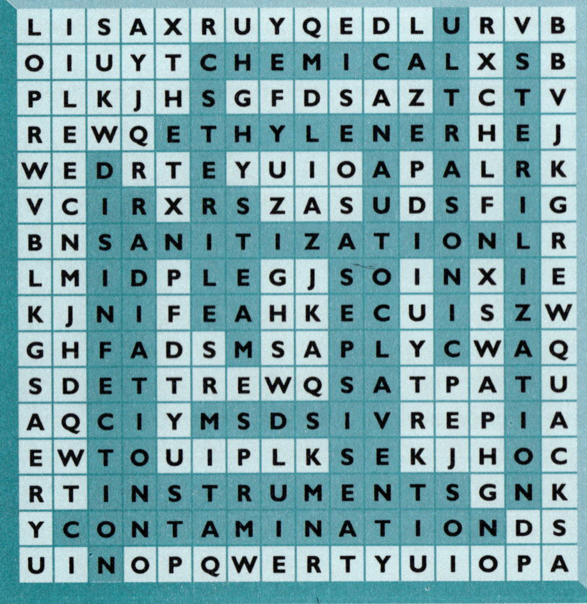

HISTORICAL HIGHLIGHTS

From ancient times, warfare created the need for some means of controlling hemorrhage and closing wounds. Egyptian writings dating back to 3000 B.C. tell of treatment of various injuries; tourniquets were used to control bleeding and wounds were sewn together with sutures.

Early records describe epidemics, purulence, fumigation, and wound management. These early concepts of infection and preventions would seem strange in light of modern scientific knowledge.

Greek surgery, as first mentioned by Homer in 1000 B.C., describes how wounds of battle were cleansed, hemorrhage was checked and then covered with compresses. Pressure, bandages, and elevation of the part was practiced by early surgeons.

Research in wound healing did not exist before the eighteenth century, when John Hunter observed and recorded for the first time some of the various patterns of healing.

The medical assistant should understand the mechanisms influencing wound healing and the negative results of hematoma, infection, wound disruption, scarring, stricture, and contracture. Wound healing is nature's way of restoring continuity and strength to injured or incised tissue.

These techniques are an important part of your function as a medical assistant.

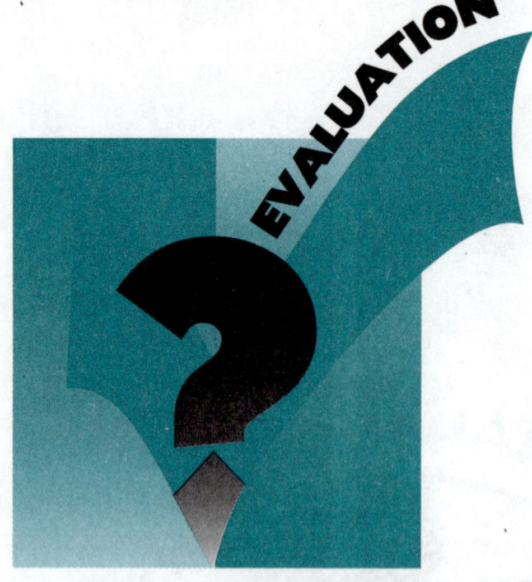

Vocabulary

Write the letter of each term on the line of its matching definition at the right.

a. surgical asepsis

b. abrasion

c. puncture

d. avulsion

e. laceration

f. incision

g. wound

h. dressing

i. bandages

j. hypoallergenic

k. Culturette

l. culture

m. Tubegauz

n. sterile field

o. mucous membranes

1. _____ a scraping away of a portion of the skin

2. _____ growth of microorganisms in special laboratory media

3. _____ a piece of gauze or other material applied to a body part as a dressing

4. _____ break in the continuity of the skin

5. _____ an irregular tear of the skin

6. _____ injury caused by tearing away a part forcibly

7. _____ substance less likely to cause an allergic reaction

8. _____ a work area prepared with sterile drapes to hold sterile supplies during a sterile procedure

9. _____ a protective covering on an injured or diseased body part

10. _____ sterile or aseptic technique

11. _____ a commercially prepared bacterial culture collection/transport system

12. _____ membrane lining passages and cavities communicating with the air

13. _____ a hole made by a sharp pointed object

14. _____ a seamless, tubular-knitted, cotton bandage, adaptable to all body parts

15. _____ a cut made with a sharp implement

Student Activities

1. Understanding additional medical terminology specific to wounds is necessary for the medical assistant who aspires to a greater understanding of this phenomena. Using a medical dictionary, look up the pronunciation and definition of the following terms and be prepared to discuss them.

    a.   adhesions
    b.   evisceration
    c.   dehiscence
    d.   gangrene
    e.   keloid
    f.   "proud flesh"

2. The Centers for Disease Control (CDC) in Atlanta, GA, recommends four surgical wound classifications: clean wounds, clean contaminated wounds, contaminated wounds, and dirty or infected wounds. Contact the CDC for its recommendations about these classifications.

Discussion Topics

1. The importance of proper wound care in the office cannot be underestimated. However, teaching patients proper wound care at home is equally as important. Discuss ways in which this can be stressed to patients.

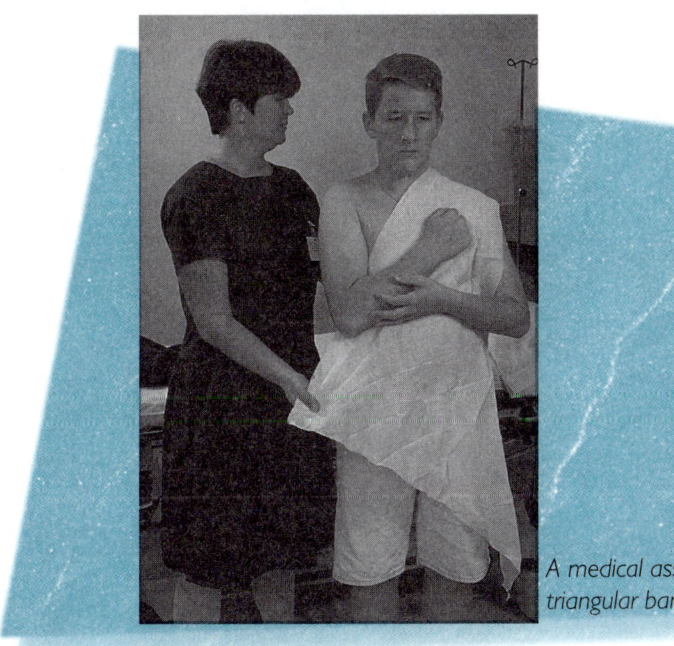

A medical assistant applies a triangular bandage.

2. Investigate ways home health agencies can be of assistance in promoting wound care by visiting and assisting patients with personal hygiene. Discuss the options and costs involved in this service.

3. Discuss the Historical Highlights and the evolution of wound care management in light of AIDS.

Review and Rationale

Answer the following questions in the space provided.

1. Why must sterile or aseptic technique be practiced?

2. Why must the outer wrapper not touch any area which is sterile?

3. Why should the final unfolding of a sterile wrapped pack be toward your body?

4. Why should you place the sterile solution cap top with the top side down?

5. Why should you cover the label of a solution bottle with the palm of your hand?

____

____

____

6. Why are sterile gloves worn?

____

____

____

7. Why do you take great precaution not to contaminate the sterile exterior of the gloves?

____

____

____

8. Why should you be careful not to allow wet items to sit on a sterile field?

____

____

____

9. Why should containers for the collection of specimens, drainage, or discharge be placed near the work area but not directly over the sterile field?

____

____

____

10. Why might it be necessary for you to steady a patient's arm, leg, or head during the operative procedure?

____

____

____

11. Why should you talk to the patient calmly?

____

____

____

12. Why should the patient be instructed not to touch or talk over the wound once it is uncovered?

____

____

____

13. Why reglove after removing a soiled dressing?

____

____

____

14. Why should tape secure the dressing, but not cover the whole dressing?

____

____

____

15. Why would you explain the surgical procedure to the patient when the physician had already done so?

____

____

____

Performance Test

In a skills laboratory, a simulation of a job-like environment, the medical assistant student must demonstrate skill and knowledge when performing the following activities without reference to source materials. Time limits for the performance of each procedure are to be assigned by the instructor.

1. Don a pair of sterile gloves, avoiding contamination, and then remove.

2. Demonstrate the proper procedure for wound care and dressing.

3. Demonstrate application of roller bandage, circular, spiral reverse, and figure eight turn bandages.

You are expected to perform the above activities with 100% accuracy 90% of the time (9 out of 10 times). If you contaminate any item during the performance of these skills, the correct actions to remedy the contaminated site must be employed 100% of the time.

Performance Checklist

DIRECTIONS: The following checklist will be used to evaluate your performance of each procedure.

Checklist 5-1: Applying and Removing Sterile Gloves

Checklist	S or NA	U	NO	Comment
1. Wash your hands.				
2. Open a glove package on a clean, dry, flat surface, with the cuff end facing you.				
3. Using your left hand, lift the right-hand glove off the wrapper by grasping the folder edge of the cuff and use it to pull the glove over your fingers and hand. (See Figure 5-1)				
4. Pick up the other glove by placing your gloved fingers straight under its cuff and lift it away from the wrapper.				
5. Pull it onto your fingers, hand, and wrist without touching your skin with the gloved hand. (See Figure 5-2)				
6. Place your gloved fingers under the cuff of the other glove and pull the remainder of the cuff over your wrist.				
7. Adjust fingers and gloves as necessary.				
8. Remove the first glove, grasp its cuff and pull it down over your hand inside out. (See Figure 5-3 A,B)				
9. Remove the other glove by reaching inside the glove cuff and pulling it off. (See Figure 5-3 C,D)				
10. Discard the gloves in an appropriate place.				

*S or NA = satisfactory or not applicable; U = unsatisfactory; NO = not observed

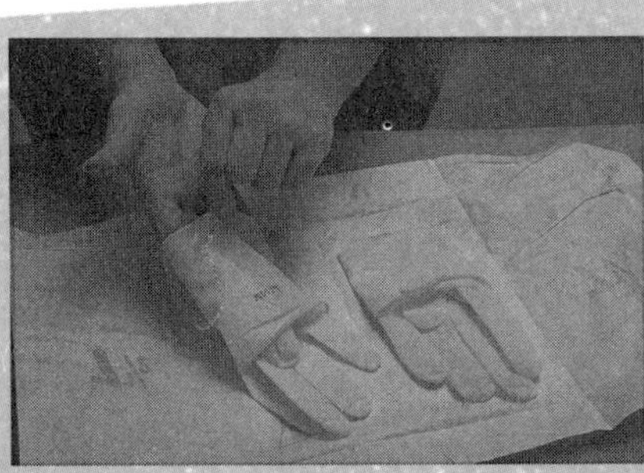

Figure 5-1 Technique for donning first sterile glove. Grasp folded edge of cuff, lift up and away from wrapper and pull onto right hand.

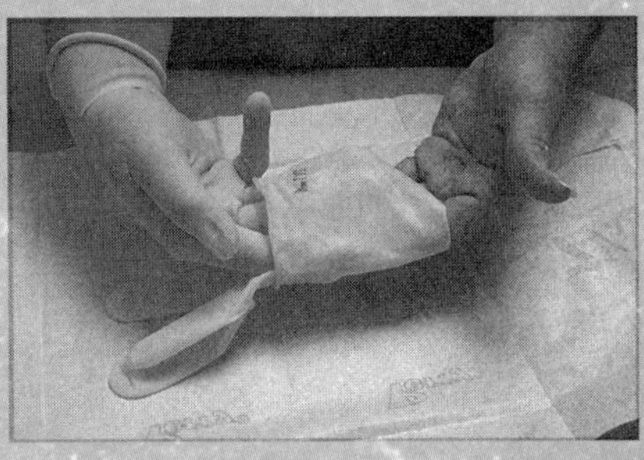

Figure 5-2 Techniques for donning second sterile glove. Place fingers of gloved hand under cuff of other glove and pull onto left hand.

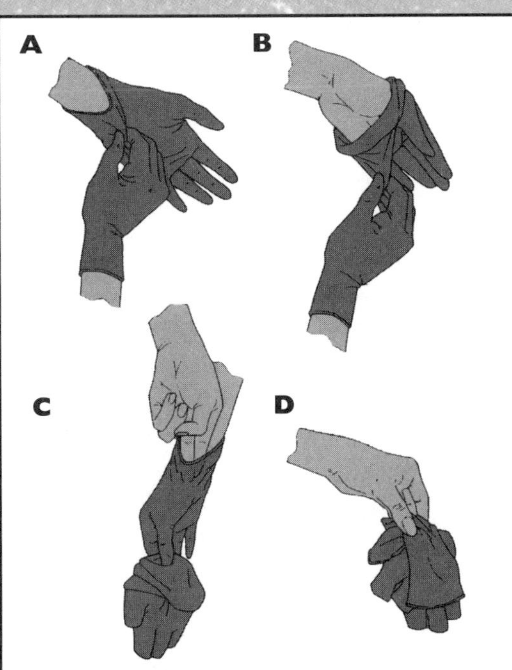

Figure 5-3 Removing gloves

A. The glove is grasped below the cuff.

B. The glove is pulled down over the hand. The glove is inside out.

C. The fingers of the ungloved hand are inserted inside the glove.

D. The glove is pulled down and over the hand and glove. The glove is inside out.

(From Sorrentino: Mosby's Textbook for Nursing Assistants 3E, St. Louis, 1992, Mosby)

Video 5: Surgical Asepsis, Sterile Technique, Minor Surgery, and Bandages

Checklist 5-2: Demonstrate wound care and dressing (See Figure 5-4)

Checklist	S or NA	U	NO	Comment
1. Wash your hands.				
2. Gather a sterile dressing tray or a prepackaged sterile dressing set: hypoallergenic tape, plastic bag for the soiled dressing, sterile disposable gloves, sterile towels and draping materials, and the laboratory requisition needed for the wound culture.				
3. Assist the patient to a relaxed, comfortable position which allows you access to the wound.				
4. Drape the patient as needed and request the patient not to touch or talk over the wound.				
5. Use aseptic techniques at all times.				
6. Use the dressing set for the sterile field.				
7. Place the plastic bag in a convenient place to receive the soiled dressing and other disposable items.				
8. Pour the antiseptic solution into the container located on the sterile field.				
9. Cut the pieces of tape to be used to secure the clean dressing.				
10. Loosen the soiled dressing and remove it with sterile forceps or a gloved hand.				
11. Check the soiled dressing for the amount and type of drainage, then discard it in the plastic bag.				
12. Observe the wound. Note location, type, and amount of drainage, pus, or necrosis. Check for an odor. Note degree of healing, and if sutures are present, note if they are intact.				
13. If infection is suspected, obtain a culture. Using a sterile applicator, obtain the specimen. Remove the sterile applicator from the sterile culture tube or Culturette.				
14. Swab the drainage area of the wound once, moving in one direction only. Place the applicator in the culture tube, secure the lid tightly and set tube aside. Remove single use exam gloves and dispose of properly.				

Continued on next page

Continued from previous page

Checklist 5-2: Demonstrate wound care and dressing (See Figure 5-4)

Checklist	S or NA	U	NO	Comment
15. Continue with wound dressing process. Put on sterile gloves using the correct procedure and pick up a gauze sponge with a hemostat or tissue forceps.				
16. Wet the sponge with the antiseptic solution.				
17. Starting at the center of the wound, stroke toward the ends using one sponge per stroke. Dispose of the sponge after each stroke.				
18. Center the sterile dressing over the wound and add layers according to the type of wound and amount of drainage.				
19. Remove gloves and dispose of them in the waste container. Set aside the reusable forceps for future sterilization.				
20. Secure the dressing with tape.				
21. Wash your hands.				
22. Attend to the patient and record the procedure and results on the patient's chart.				
23. Label culture tubes or Culturettes completely and accurately.				
24. Attach a completed lab requisition and send the culture to the laboratory.				
25. Attend to the treatment room as needed.				

*S or NA = satisfactory or not applicable; U = unsatisfactory; NO = not observed

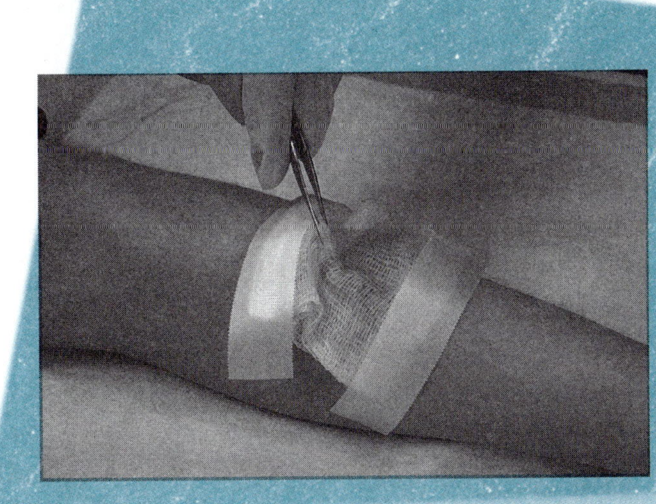

Figure 5-4
Removing soiled dressing with a forceps.

Checklist 5-3: Demonstrate use of bandages: roller bandage demonstrating circular turn (Figure 5-5)

Checklist	S or NA	U	NO	Comment
1. Wrap the roller bandage by placing the end portion of the bias next to the patient's skin, anchoring the bandage at the start and end of the procedure.				
2. Circle the bandage around the body part, allowing a corner edge to jut out.				
3. Fold the edge down over the first turn and cover with the second circular turn of the bandage.				

*S or NA = satisfactory or not applicable; U = unsatisfactory; NO = not observed

Figure 5-5

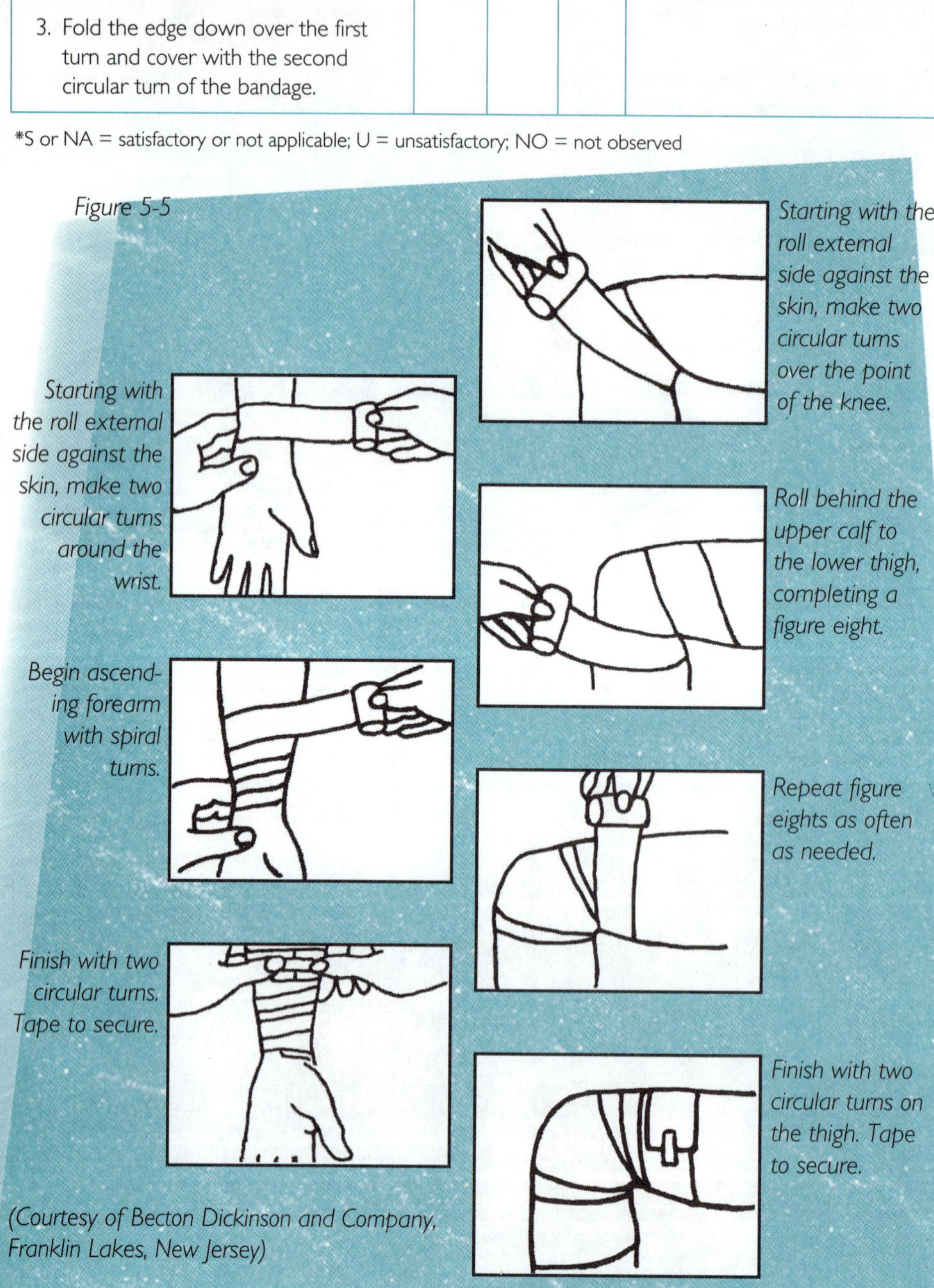

(Courtesy of Becton Dickinson and Company, Franklin Lakes, New Jersey)

Checklist 5-4: Demonstrate use of bandages: roller bandage demonstrating spiral-reverse turn (See Figure 5-5)

Checklist	S or NA	U	NO	Comment
1. Wrap the roller bandage by angling each circling of the bandage so that every turn overlaps the previous one by $1/3$ to $1/2$ the width of the bandage.				

*S or NA = satisfactory or not applicable; U = unsatisfactory; NO = not observed

Checklist 5-5: Demonstrate use of bandages: roller bandage demonstrating figure eight turn (See Figure 5-5)

Checklist	S or NA	U	NO	Comment
1. Turn the roller bandage at a diagonal to alternately ascend and descend the area, making a figure eight around the part.				

*S or NA = satisfactory or not applicable; U = unsatisfactory; NO = not observed

Multiple Choice

From the options listed under each question or statement, select the correct answer or answers. Write the corresponding letter or letters in the answer space.

1. To open a peel-down package: _______
   a. unfold the flaps away from you
   b. pull evenly downward along sealed edges
   c. use sterile scissors to edge off top and pull out contents from the cut edge
   d. none of the above

2. Which of the following should you use to organize sterile equipment and supplies? _______
   a. sterile transfer forceps
   b. sterile gloves
   c. a or b
   d. none of the above

3. Why is it important to use aseptic techniques when pouring a sterile solution? _______
   a. solutions are drugs
   b. OSHA requirement
   c. MSDA suggested procedure
   d. all of the above

4. Assisting the physician with minor surgical procedures, your responsibilities include: _______
   a. readying the room and supplies
   b. preparing the patient both physically and mentally
   c. assisting the physician as needed
   d. all of the above

5. What will happen when wet items are allowed to sit on a sterile field? _______
   a. the patient will see it
   b. contamination
   c. nothing
   d. chemical reaction to the basin

6. Any physical injury involving a break in external or internal soft body parts is called a: _______
   a. laceration
   b. evisceration
   c. injury
   d. wound

7. First intention is when the: _______
   a. antibiotic first selected has the greatest potential for eradicating the infection
   b. wound edges cannot be brought together
   c. edges of wounds can be brought together
   d. wound has extensive tissue loss or damage

8. Materials placed directly over wounds are called: _______
   a. Tubegauz
   b. Culturette
   c. dressings
   d. bandages

9. What holds dressings in place? _______
   a. hypoallergenic cloth and paper tape
   b. transparent tape
   c. elastic cloth tape and adhesive tape
   d. all of the above

10. One of the following is not a characteristic of elastic or gauze bandage: _______
    a. economical
    b. absorbent
    c. porous and allows air to reach the wound
    d. nonadhering

11. Seamless, tubular-knitted, cotton bandages conforming to all body areas are called: _______
    a. Webril
    b. Tubegauz
    c. Tubex
    d. Esmarch

12. Which turn is used for anchoring bandages at the start and end of any wrapping procedure and is used on body parts which are even in size? _______
    a. circular
    b. spiral
    c. spiral-reverse
    d. figure eight

13. The recurrent turn is used to bandage: _______
    a. wrist, elbow, ankle or knee
    b. leg, thigh, or forearm
    c. head, fingers, or toes
    d. none of the above

14. Bandages are used to: _______
    a. hold dressings or splints in place
    b. immobilize or support body parts
    c. protect an injured body part
    d. apply pressure over an area
    e. all of the above

15. Observe the wound and note the: _______
    a. location and type
    b. odor
    c. amount of drainage, pus, or necrosis
    d. all of the above
    e. none of the above

True or False

Determine whether each of the following statements is true or false. Check the box marked T or F at the left of the statement.

T   F

☐ ☐ 1. When performing procedures in which normally sterile body parts are entered, the body is highly susceptible to infection.

☐ ☐ 2. Proper surgical asepsis assures that an area and the supplies in that area are kept sterile throughout a procedure.

☐ ☐ 3. The outer wrapper of a surgical package creates a sterile field.

☐ ☐ 4. To open a peel-down package, pull evenly downward along sealed edges.

☐ ☐ 5. Use individually wrapped sterile transfer forceps for each procedure.

☐ ☐ 6. When removing a cap from a sterile solution, be sure to place it on a level surface with the top side up.

☐ ☐ 7. If either glove tears, remove and discard the torn glove and replace with a new one.

☐ ☐ 8. All laboratories require an anaerobic Culturette be used for specimen collection.

☐ ☐ 9. Triangular bandages are large pieces of cloth used as arm slings.

☐ ☐ 10. Tubegauz are elastic bandages made of woven cotton used to bandage areas requiring firm support.

Word Puzzle

Complete the puzzle using the following medical terminology definitions related to surgical asepsis, sterile technique, minor surgery, and bandages.

ACROSS

3. two surfaces holding together
4. injury caused by tearing away a part forcibly
5. a protective covering on an injured or diseased body part
7. bursting open, as a surgical wound
8. a mass of excessive granulation

DOWN

1. scar formation of the skin
2. a piece of gauze or other material applied to a body part as a dressing
4. a scraping away of a portion of the skin
6. spilling out of abdominal contents

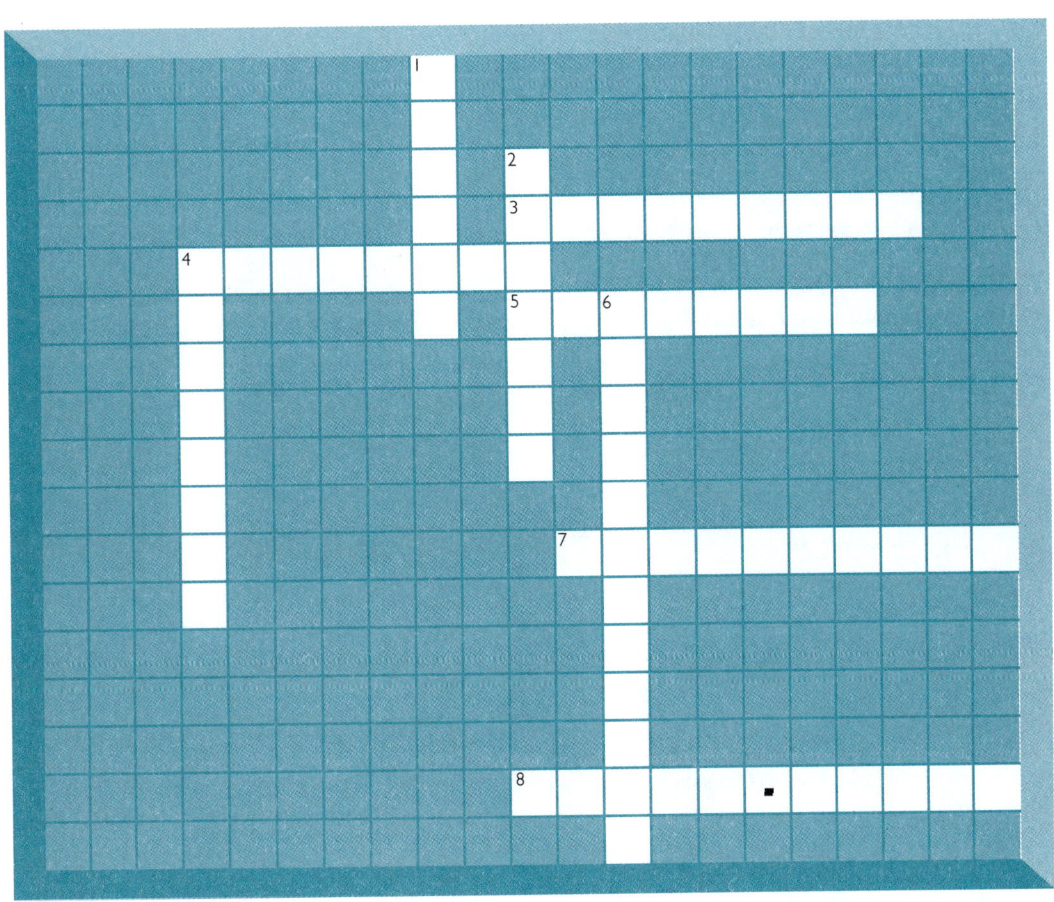

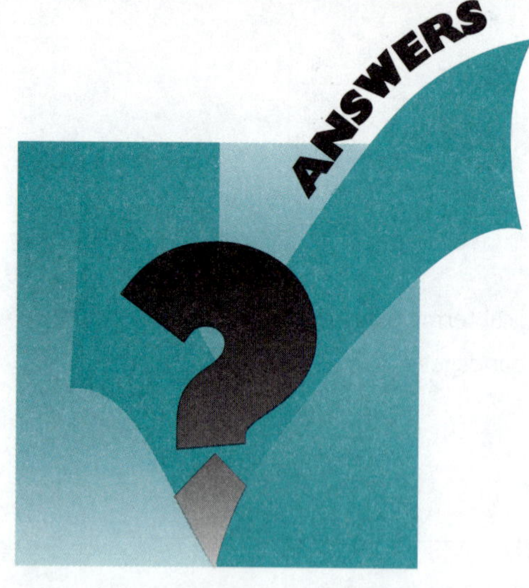

Vocabulary

1. b	4. g	7. j	10. a	13. c
2. l	5. e	8. n	11. k	14. m
3. i	6. d	9. h	12 o	15. f

Student Activities

1. a. adhesions - two surfaces holding together

   b. evisceration - spilling out of abdominal contents

   c. dehiscence - bursting open, as a surgical wound

   d. gangrene - necrosis or death of tissue

   e. keloid - scar formation of the skin

   f. "proud flesh" - a mass of excessive granulation tissue when a wound shows no other sign of healing

2. Answers may vary.

Discussion Topics

1–3. Answers may vary.

Review and Rationale

1. To reduce the chances of infection, surgical asepsis, often called sterile or aseptic technique, must be practiced.

2. The outer wrapper is not sterile and must not touch any area which is sterile.

3. The final unfolding of a sterile pack toward you will keep you from reaching over the sterile field.

4. To prevent contamination, hold the cap top in your hand and place it on a level surface with the top side down.

5. Cover the label with the palm of your hand to keep it from being soiled in case of spillage.

6. Sterile gloves are worn to protect you and the patient from infection and to safely handle sterile supplies and equipment.

7. Hands are the greatest source of contamination so take great precaution not to contaminate the sterile exterior of the gloves.

8. Do not allow wet items to sit on a sterile field because contamination will result.

9. These containers should be placed near the work area for convenience, but not directly over the sterile field as these items may contaminate the field.

10. It may be necessary for you to steady a patient's arm, leg, or head so that abrupt movements are avoided during the operative procedure.

11. Talking to the patient calmly may relax the patient and distract him/her from pain or discomfort.

12. Once it is uncovered microorganisms can spread to the area.

13. The gloves used for loosening and removing the dressing are now contaminated and must be discarded.

14. The tape should not cover the whole dressing, as this would interfere with air circulation.

15. The medical assistant usually briefly explains the procedure again on the day of the surgery to answer questions and help the patient relax.

Multiple Choice

1. b	4. d	7. c	10. a	13. c
2. c	5. b	8. c	11. b	14. e
3. a	6. d	9. d	12. a	15. d

True or False

1. T	3. F	5. T	7. F	9. T
2. T	4. T	6. F	8. F	10. F

Word Puzzle

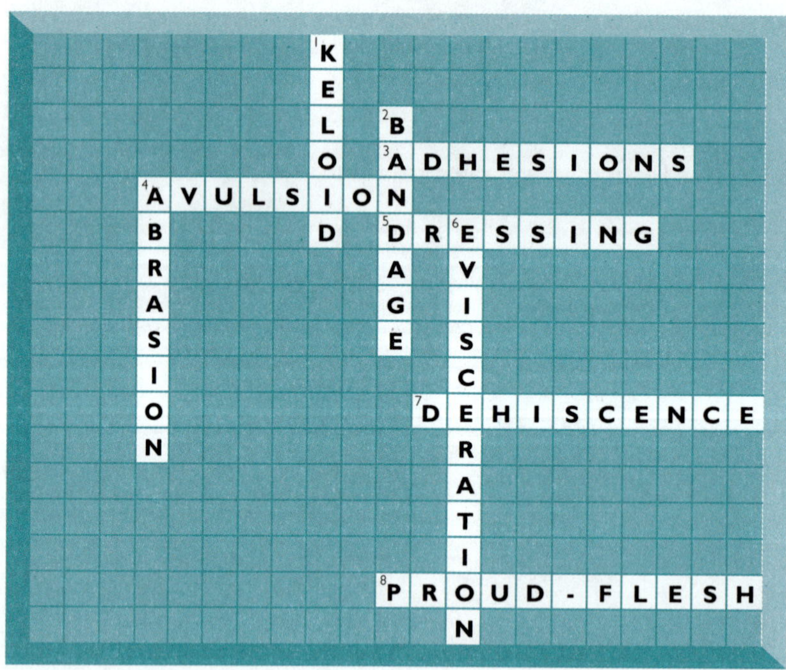

HISTORICAL HIGHLIGHTS

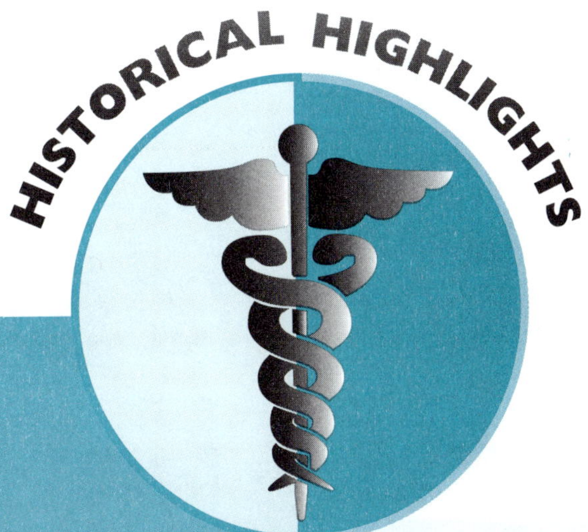

The German physician Robert Koch was the founder of bacteriology and won a Nobel prize for isolating the tubercle bacillus. **Bacteriology** is the science dealing with micro-organisms.

Dr. Koch defined these four assumptions:

1. A specific organism must be seen in all cases of an infectious disease.

2. This organism must be obtained in pure culture.

3. Organisms from pure cultures must reproduce the disease in experimental animals.

4. The organism must be recoverable from the experimental animals.

These assumptions serve as guides to the discovery of agents causing many diseases.

Identification of a pathogenic organism which may be causing a disease process is the first step in treating the disease. Observance of the prescribed techniques for obtaining cultures, proper patient education and instruction, and prompt collecting and handling of specimens is an important part of your medical assistant skills.

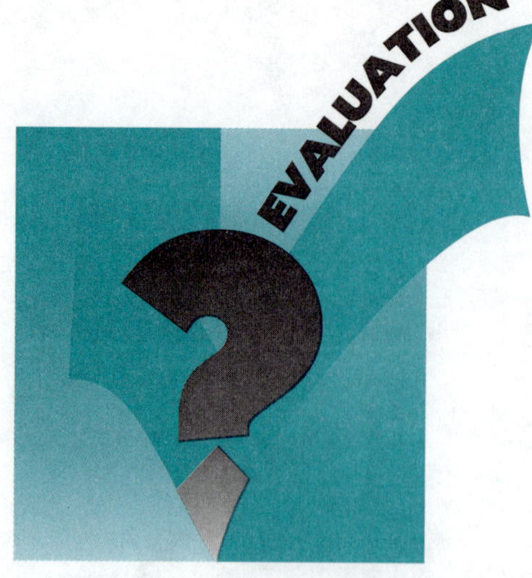

Vocabulary

Write the letter of each term on the line of its matching definition at the right.

a. specimens

b. urinalysis

c. random specimen

d. clean catch specimen

e. 24-hour urine specimen

f. stool specimen

g. Hemoccult

h. sputum specimen

i. expectorate

j. throat culture

k. occult

l. pharynx

m. larynx

n. cytology

o. bacteriology

1. _______ windpipe

2. _______ collection of urine following the first, early morning voiding

3. _______ hidden

4. _______ test to determine the presence of infectious organisms

5. _______ urine voided at any time of the day or night and collected from any portion of the urine flow

6. _______ specimen taken to determine the presence and type of microscopic organisms causing an infection

7. _______ specimen to diagnose presence of parasites and ova, blood, infectious diseases, and various metabolism disorders

8. _______ body fluids, secretions, excretions or tissue removed from a patient's body for laboratory tests

9. _______ study of cells

10. _______ urine specimen with limited contamination by skin bacteria

11. _______ study of bacteria

12. _______ determination of how the kidneys are functioning

13. _______ throat

14. _______ removal of secretions of the respiratory tract

15. _______ test for detecting the presence of occult blood in fecal matter

Student Activities

1. Different specimens require different fixatives. Contact several local vendors of laboratory supplies for information about the newest products available. How do they vary? Are there any common, less expensive methods of fixing specimens?

2. Arrange a visit to a laboratory in a family practice office to observe specimen collection procedures and processing.

3. Do you know how important it is for the office laboratory to be proficient in its testing program? If it is competent or proficient, how do you know the results obtained from the lab are accurate? Contact several offices in your community and ask what proficiency testing program* they use. Contact a medical evaluation laboratory for information about its service.

*Proficiency testing is the practice of testing specimens of unknown value provided by an external source as a means to assure accurate lab testing. It is part of a comprehensive program to meet legal requirements.

Discussion Topics

1. Collecting urine specimens from children and adults who can understand spoken or written directions is not as complicated as collecting a much needed specimen from an infant or toddler. Discuss ways in which you can collect urine specimens from these challenging patients: a 2-month-old and 7-month-old child.

2. How safe are the gloves you wear? How do you know if they are defective? What if it

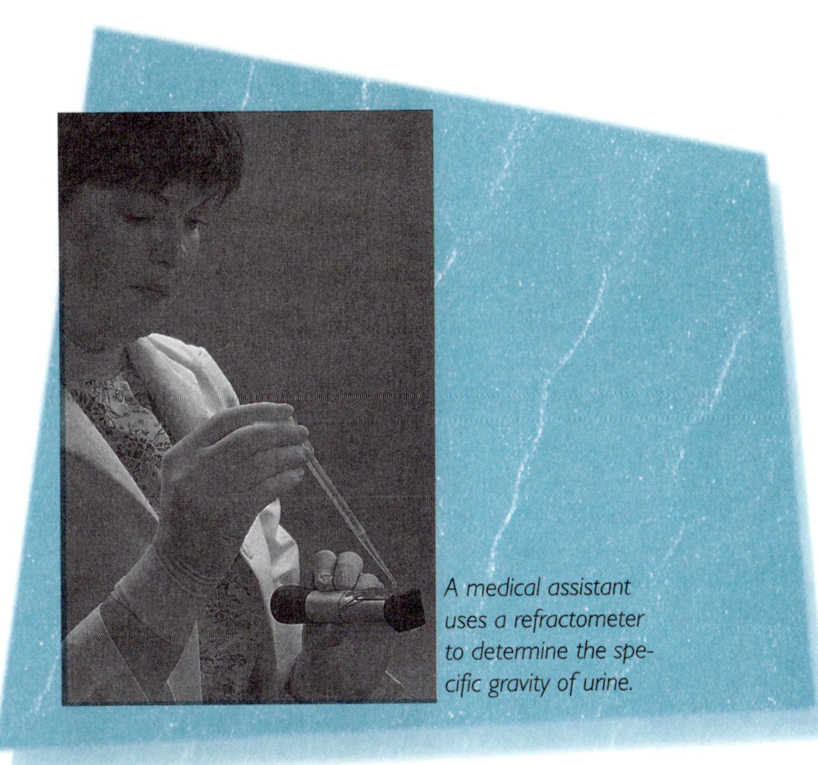

A medical assistant uses a refractometer to determine the specific gravity of urine.

has pinholes? Who inspects gloves? Who establishes guidelines for testing gloves? These questions and others you can think of should spark a desire to be cautious about the purchase and dependability of gloves. How do you find the answers to these questions?

Review and Rationale

Answer the following questions in the space provided.

1. Why is it important to ask the patient if he/she is on a special diet or taking any medications prior to performing a urinalysis?

____

____

____

2. Why should the patient empty his/her bladder first before collecting a stool specimen?

____

____

____

3. Why should the tongue depressor or spatula used in obtaining a stool specimen not be disposed of in the wastebasket?

____

____

____

4. Prior to giving a specimen, why should patients avoid foods such as: red meat, turnips, and melons as well as drugs such as aspirin, iron tablets, and vitamin C in excess of 250 milligrams per day?

____

____

____

5. What does saying "ah" do when obtaining a throat culture?

____

____

____

6. Why should the tongue blade be placed over two-thirds of the patient's extended tongue and depressed?

____

____

____

7. Why should you spray the cytology smear within four seconds of making it?

____

____

____

8. Why do you pass the cytology slide quickly through the flame of the Bunsen burner and repeat the motion three or four times to heat fix the slide?

____

____

____

9. Why is the coverglass placed over the saline and the cytology specimen?

____

____

____

10. Why is it important to send the specimen in the transport container to the lab immediately?

____

____

____

Performance Test

In a skills laboratory, a simulation of a job-like environment, the medical assistant student must demonstrate skill and knowledge in performing the following procedures without reference to source materials. You will need a person to play the role of the patient. Time limits for the performance of each procedure are to be assigned by the instructor.

1. Demonstrate proficiency in instructing patient to collect urine specimens in each of the following methods:
   a. random specimen
   b. midstream specimen
   c. clean catch specimen
   d. 24-hour specimen

2. Demonstrate proficiency in instructing patient to collect stool specimens.
   a. Perform Hemoccult Slide Test

3. Describe the process for acquiring the following specimens:
   a. sputum specimen
   b. throat culture
   c. nasopharyngeal culture

4. Describe methods for obtaining the following smears:
   a. cytology smear
   b. bacteriology smear
   c. vaginal smear and culture

You are expected to perform these activities with 100% accuracy 90% of the time (9 out of 10 times).

Performance Checklist

DIRECTIONS: The following checklist will be used to evaluate your performance of each procedure.

Checklist 6-1: Collection of a Random Urine Specimen. Instruct patient in obtaining a random urine specimen:

Checklist	S or NA	U	NO	Comment
1. Wash hands.				
2. Assemble equipment.				
3. Introduce yourself and identify the patient.				
4. Explain the procedure.				
5. Follow Universal Precautions.				
6. Provide the patient with a sterile wide-mouthed container and explain how much urine should be voided into the container.				
7. Receive specimen from patient.				
8. Label specimen and complete the laboratory requisition.				
9. Wash your hands.				
10. Record the procedure on the patient's chart.				
11. Discard used supplies and contaminated items appropriately.				

*S or NA = satisfactory or not applicable; U = unsatisfactory; NO = not observed

Checklist 6-2: Collection of a Midstream Specimen. This specimen is collected from the middle of the urine flow. Instruct patient in obtaining a midstream urine specimen:

Checklist	S or NA	U	NO	Comment
1. Wash hands.				
2. Assemble equipment.				
3. Introduce yourself and identify the patient.				
4. Explain the procedure.				
5. Follow Universal Precautions.				
6. Instruct patient to begin voiding process and then without stopping, collect a portion of the urine from the middle of the urine flow into the clean container.				
7. Instruct patient to void last part of the urine flow into the toilet.				
8. Receive specimen from patient.				
9. Label specimen and complete the laboratory requisition.				
10. Wash your hands.				
11. Record the procedure on the patient's chart.				
12. Discard used supplies and contaminated items appropriately.				

*S or NA = satisfactory or not applicable; U = unsatisfactory; NO = not observed

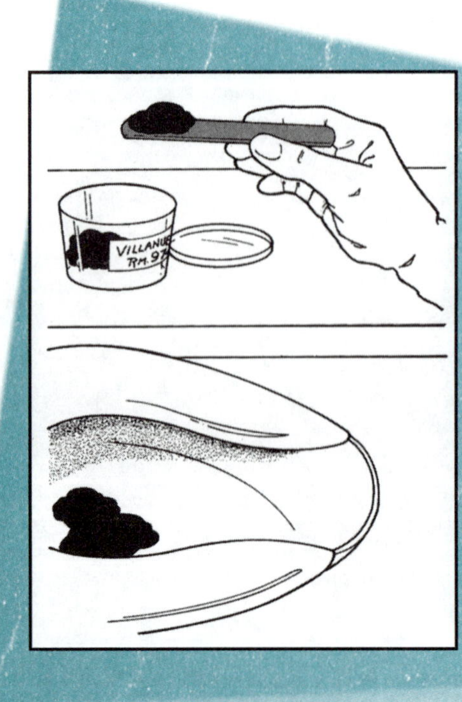

Figure 6-1 A tongue blade is used to transfer a small amount of stool from the bedpan to the specimen container. (From Sorrentino: Mosby's Textbook for Nursing Assistants 3E, St. Louis, 1992, Mosby)

Checklist 6-3: Collection of a Clean-Catch Urine Specimen.   This is a specimen with limited contamination by skin bacteria. Instruct the patient in obtaining a clean catch urine specimen:

Checklist	S or NA	U	NO	Comment
1. Wash hands.				
2. Assemble equipment.				
3. Introduce yourself and identify the patient.				
4. Explain the procedure.				
5. Follow Universal Precautions.				
6. Instruct patient to wash the external genitalia with soap and water or a mild antiseptic towel.				
7. Supply patient with clean, dry container or a sterile container.				
8. Instruct patient to void using the midstream collection method.				
9. Receive specimen from patient.				
10. Label specimen and complete the laboratory requisition.				
11. Record the procedure on the patient's chart.				
12. Discard used supplies and contaminated items appropriately.				

Checklist 6-4: 24-Hour Urine Specimen. This specimen is collected for 24 hours following the first, early morning voiding. Instruct patient in collecting 24-hour urine specimen:

Checklist	S or NA	U	NO	Comment
1. Wash hands.				
2. Assemble equipment.				
3. Introduce yourself and identify the patient.				
4. Explain the procedure.				
5. Follow Universal Precautions.				
6. Instruct patient to collect all urine for a 24-hour period following the first, early morning voiding.				
7. Receive specimen from patient.				
8. Label specimen and complete the laboratory requisition.				
9. Wash hands.				
10. Record the procedure on the patient's chart.				
11. Discard used supplies and contaminated items appropriately.				

*S or NA = satisfactory or not applicable; U = unsatisfactory; NO = not observed

Checklist 6-5: Stool Specimen (See Figure 6-1) Instruct patient in collection of a stool specimen:

Checklist	S or NA	U	NO	Comment
1. Wash hands.				
2. Assemble equipment.				
3. Introduce yourself and identify the patient.				
4. Explain the procedure.				
5. Follow Universal Precautions.				
6. Instruct patient to use bedpan or specimen container to deposit stool.				
7. Receive the specimen, cover it, and label it with the patient's name, date, and time.				
8. Take it to your work area.				
9. With gloved hands, using tongue depressor or spatula, transfer one to two teaspoons of the stool into the specimen container.				
10. Place or smear the specimen only on the inside of the container.				
11. Place the lid securely on the container.				
12. Deposit the tongue depressor or spatula in the paper bag and wrap it securely for proper disposal.				
13. Observe color and consistency of the feces and report any abnormalities.				
14. Empty and clean the bedpan.				
15. Wash hands.				
16. Label specimen container and attach correct, completed laboratory requisition.				
17. Send or take labeled specimen to the laboratory immediately.				
18. Wash your hands.				
19. Record the procedure on the patient's chart.				

*S or NA = satisfactory or not applicable; U = unsatisfactory; NO = not observed

Checklist 6-6: Hemoccult Slide Test. Instruct patient and perform a Hemoccult Slide Test:

Checklist	S or NA	U	NO	Comment
1. Instruct patient on special diet two days prior to exam. Avoid food such as rare, red meat, turnips, and melons. Refrain from taking drugs such as aspirin, iron tablets, and vitamin C in excess of 250 mg per day.				
2. Instruct patient in stool specimen preparation.				
3. Wash hands.				
4. Assemble equipment:				
a. patient's stool specimen container				
b. specimen applicator				
c. patient Hemoccult envelope with an identification card				
d. Hemoccult developer.				
5. Follow Universal Precautions.				
6. Receive specimen from patient.				
7. Label specimen container with patient's name.				
8. On envelope identification card, write the patient's name, age, address, phone number, and date the specimen is collected.				
9. Open the identification flap. With one end of the applicator, collect a small sample of stool. Apply a thin smear inside box A.				
10. Reuse the applicator to obtain a second sample from a different part of the stool specimen and apply a thin smear inside of box B.				
11. Close the cover and discard the applicator in appropriate waste container.				
12. Open back flap of the slide, noting fecal-smear A and B boxes and the positive and negative performance monitor.				
13. Apply one drop only of Hemoccult developer between the positive and negative performance monitor and read results within ten seconds.				
14. Apply two drops of Hemoccult developer to the paper directly over each smear box and read the results within 60 seconds.				
15. Wash hands.				
16. Record results on patient's chart.				

*S or NA = satisfactory or not applicable; U = unsatisfactory; NO = not observed

Checklist 6-7: Sputum Specimen Collection.

Checklist	S or NA	U	NO	Comment
1. Wash hands.				
2. Assemble equipment:				
a. sterile specimen container				
b. label				
c. laboratory requisition				
d. paper bag and tape				
3. Introduce yourself and identify the patient.				
4. Explain the procedure.				
5. Follow Universal Precautions.				
6. Give the sterile specimen container to the patient and ask that he/she not touch the inside of the container.				
7. Instruct the patient to cough deeply and expectorate directly into the container. (Figure 6-2)				
8. Label the container accurately and completely and indicate required tests on the laboratory requisition.				
9. Secure the sputum container lid with tape and place the container in a paper bag.				
10. Then attach the laboratory requisition and send the specimen to the lab.				
11. Wash your hands and record information and your observations on the patient's chart.				

*S or NA = satisfactory or not applicable; U = unsatisfactory; NO = not observed

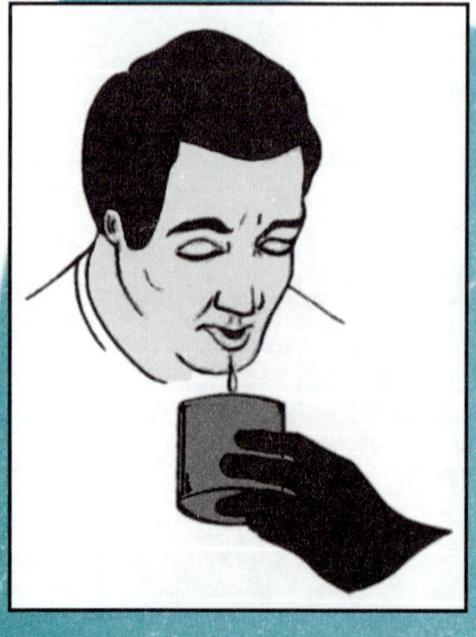

Figure 6-2 The patient expectorates directly into the center of the specimen container. (From Sorrentino: Mosby's Textbook for Nursing Assistants 3/E, St. Louis,, 1992, Mosby)

Checklist 6-8: Throat Culture Specimen Collection

Checklist	S or NA	U	NO	Comment
1. Wash hands.				
2. Assemble equipment: a. sterile cotton-tipped applicator b. sterile tube or Culturette c. clean tongue depressor d. label e. laboratory requisition.				
3. Introduce yourself and identify the patient.				
4. Explain the procedure.				
5. Follow Universal Precautions.				
6. Ask patient to sit upright, facing you.				
7. Make sure the area in which you are working is well lighted.				
8. Remove the sterile cotton-tipped applicator from the culture or Culturette tube.				
9. Ask the patient to open his/her mouth as wide as possible, extend the tongue, and say "ah."				
10. Place the tongue blade over two-thirds of the patient's extended tongue and depress.				
11. With the cotton-tipped applicator, swab the area at the very back of the throat on both sides. (Special attention should be taken to swab any red, raw, or pus coated areas.)				
12. Remove the applicator and the tongue blade and place the applicator in the culture or Culturette tube.				
13. Secure the lid then discard the tongue blade in a covered waste container.				
14. If the applicator is placed in a Culturette, release the transport medium by crushing the ampule with your fingers at the designated place.				
15. Wash your hands.				
16. Label the culture tube.				
17. Attach the requisitions and send the culture tube to the lab.				
18. Record the procedure on the patient's chart.				
19. Discard used supplies and contaminated items appropriately.				

*S or NA = satisfactory or not applicable; U = unsatisfactory; NO = not observed

Checklist 6-9: Nasopharyngeal Culture Specimen Collection

Checklist	S or NA	U	NO	Comment
1. Wash hands.				
2. Assemble equipment:				
a. sterile cotton-tipped applicator in a sterile tube or Culturette				
b. label				
c. laboratory requisition				
3. Introduce yourself and identify the patient.				
4. Explain the procedure.				
5. Follow Universal Precautions.				
6. Insert a sterile cotton-tipped applicator through the nose and into the nasopharyngeal area.				
7. Gently rotate the applicator to obtain the specimen.				
8. Remove the applicator, and place it into the sterile culture tube.				
9. Secure the lid, label the specimen, and send it to the lab with the correct laboratory requisition.				
10. Record the procedure on the patient's chart.				

*S or NA = satisfactory or not applicable; U = unsatisfactory; NO = not observed

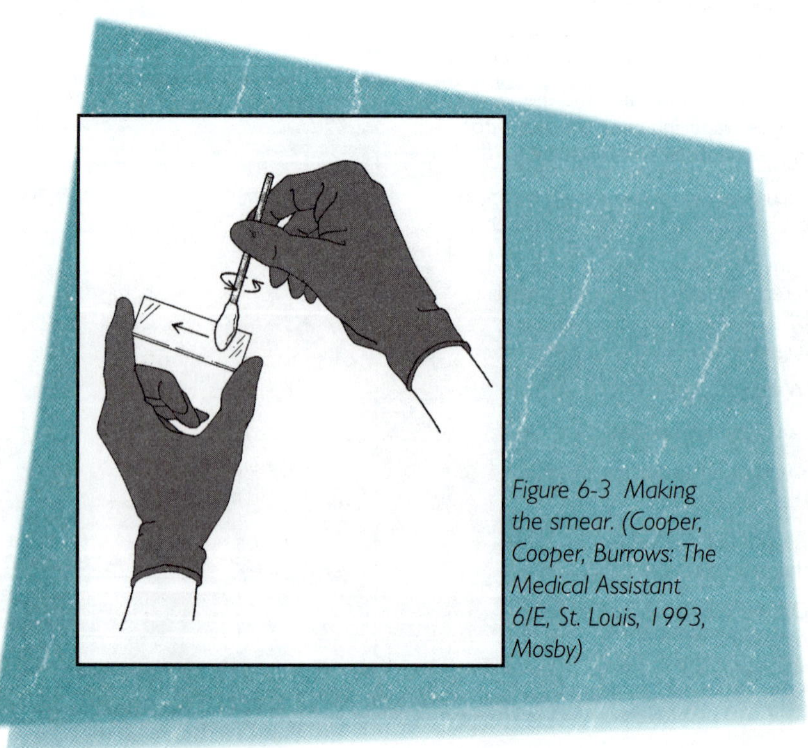

Figure 6-3 Making the smear. (Cooper, Cooper, Burrows: The Medical Assistant 6/E, St. Louis, 1993, Mosby)

Checklist 6-10: Describe Methods for Obtaining Cytology and Bacteriology Smears (See Figure 6-3)

Checklist	S or NA	U	NO	Comment
1. Wash hands.				
2. Assemble equipment:				
a. sterile cotton-tipped applicator				
b. frosted-end glass slide				
c. fixture spray such as Cyto-Fix				
d. cardboard or plastic slide holder				
e. laboratory requisition				
3. Write patient's name and date on the frosted end of the slide.				
4. Take the applicator with your dominant hand, grasping the distal end of the stick.				
5. Hold the glass slide between the thumb and index finger of your nondominant hand.				
6. Spread the specimen across the slide, rotating the applicator in the opposite direction using correct motion.				
7. Discard contaminated applicator tip in a covered waste container.				
Slide Fixing Process for Cytology Smear:				
8. Fix the smear by immediately spraying it with the fixture spray.				
9. Spray the slide with a continuous flow, from left to right and then right to left.				
10. Allow the slide to dry for four to six minutes.				
11. Wash hands.				
12. Place the cytology slide in a designated plastic or cardboard container, label it, and attach the laboratory requisition and send it to the laboratory.				
Slide Fixing Process for Bacteriology Smear:				
8. Place the smear on a flat surface and allow it to air dry for approximately one half hour.				
9. Using the slide forceps, pass the slide quickly through the flame of the Bunsen burner. Repeat this motion three or four times to heat fix the slide.				
10. Wash hands.				
11. Place the bacteriology slide in a designated plastic or cardboard container, label it, and attach the laboratory requisition and send it to the laboratory.				

*S or NA = satisfactory or not applicable; U = unsatisfactory; NO = not observed

Checklist 6-11: Describe Methods for Obtaining a Vaginal Smear and Culture for Trichomoniasis Vaginitis.

Checklist	S or NA	U	NO	Comment
1. Wash hands.				
2. Assemble equipment:				
a. cotton-tipped applicator with which to take specimen sample				
b. small amount of normal saline solution				
c. slide with a depressed section in the middle				
d. coverglass.				
3. Introduce yourself and identify the patient.				
4. Explain the procedure.				
5. Follow Universal Precautions.				
6. While assisting the physician with a pelvic exam, place a small amount of normal saline in the depressed, middle area of the slide.				
7. Receive specimen from the physician and dip the saturated applicator into the saline solution on the slide.				
8. Discard the applicator in a covered waste container.				
9. Place the coverglass over the saline and the specimen in the depressed middle section of the slide.				
10. Place the specimen in the transport container, attach the laboratory requisition, and send the smear to the lab at once.				
11. Discard used supplies and contaminated items appropriately.				
12. Wash hands.				
13. Record the procedure on the patient's chart.				

*S or NA = satisfactory or not applicable; U = unsatisfactory; NO = not observed

Multiple Choice

From the options listed under each question or statement, select the correct answer or answers. Write the corresponding letter or letters in the answer space.

1. Laboratory tests provide a means for: _________
   a. evaluating a patient's health status
   b. identifying pathogenic organisms
   c. treatment methods
   d. a and b
   e. none of the above

2. All except one of the following are the most common urine specimens the physician may order: _________
   a. random specimen
   b. catheter specimen
   c. clean catch specimen
   d. 24-hour specimen
   e. midstream specimen

3. Which urine specimen is described as urine voided at any time of the day or night and collected from any portion of the urine flow? _________
   a. clean catch urine specimen
   b. midstream urine specimen
   c. 24-hour urine specimen
   d. any of the above
   e. a or b

4. Stool specimens help diagnose the presence of: _________
   a. parasites or ova
   b. blood
   c. infectious diseases
   d. various metabolism disorders
   e. all of the above

5. Patients are placed on a special diet when stool is examined for: _________
   a. fecal blood
   b. Hemoccult
   c. parasites
   d. infectious diseases

6. What does the following physician's order mean: "sputum culture × 3"? ________
   a. schedule patient for three o'clock appointment
   b. collect three different specimens at three different times
   c. collect one specimen and divide it into three different containers
   d. none of the above

7. When instructing the patient to *expectorate* directly into the container, what does the italicized word mean? ________
   a. vomit
   b. belch
   c. bring forth secretions of the respiratory tract
   d. cough

8. Throat cultures are performed to determine the presence and type of microscopic organisms causing: ________
   a. strep throat
   b. whooping cough
   c. diphtheria
   d. all of the above

9. To perform a throat culture, which of the following is not required? ________
   a. sterile cotton-tipped applicator
   b. saline solution
   c. sterile tube or Culturette
   d. clean tongue depressor

10. Which procedure is performed on infants suspected of having whooping cough, pneumonia, or croup? ________
    a. urine culture
    b. blood culture
    c. nasopharyngeal culture
    d. sputum specimen

11. Types of cytology or bacteriology smears for laboratory examination include all of the following except: ________
    a. blood
    b. bronchial fluids
    c. cyst fluid
    d. urine

12. Passing the bacteriology slide through the Bunsen burner: ________
    a. prepares it for the fixture spray
    b. attaches the microorganisms to the slide
    c. distorts the cells
    d. helps release cells so they wash off the slide easier

13. Gynecological conditions are diagnosed by: _________
    a. vaginal and cervical smears
    b. 24-hour urine collection specimen
    c. test for occult blood
    d. none of the above

14. What type of slide is used for a vaginal smear to detect trichomoniasis vaginitis? _________
    a. one with a depressed section in the middle and a coverglass
    b. frosted-tipped slide
    c. clear glass slide
    d. slide with a coverglass

15. What can be used in place of a sterile cotton-tipped applicator in a sterile tube? _________
    a. Cyto-Fix
    b. Q-tip applicator
    c. Culturette
    d. Hemoccult slide

True or False

Determine whether each of the following statements is true or false. Check the box marked T or F at the left of the statement.

T F

☐ ☐ 1. Laboratory tests can be performed on all body specimens.

☐ ☐ 2. Treatment methods can be administered once the cause of a disease process is identified.

☐ ☐ 3. Saying "ah" maximizes the gag reflex.

☐ ☐ 4. The fixing process for cytology and bacteriology smears are the same.

☐ ☐ 5. The PAP smear is the most common vaginal and cervical smear taken.

☐ ☐ 6. If a trichomonas organism is present, it must be viewed and identified within 24 hours.

☐ ☐ 7. Urinalysis can be affected by diet and medications.

☐ ☐ 8. To fix cytology smears pass slide quickly through the flame of the Bunsen burner.

T   F

☐ ☐   9. The Hemoccult slide test detects the presence of occult blood in fecal matter.

☐ ☐   10. To fix bacteriology smears, spray them with the fixture spray.

Word Puzzle

Circle the following medical terms related to collecting and handling specimens.

specimens	occult	organism
expectorate	random	secretions
larynx	urinalysis	
cytology	culture	

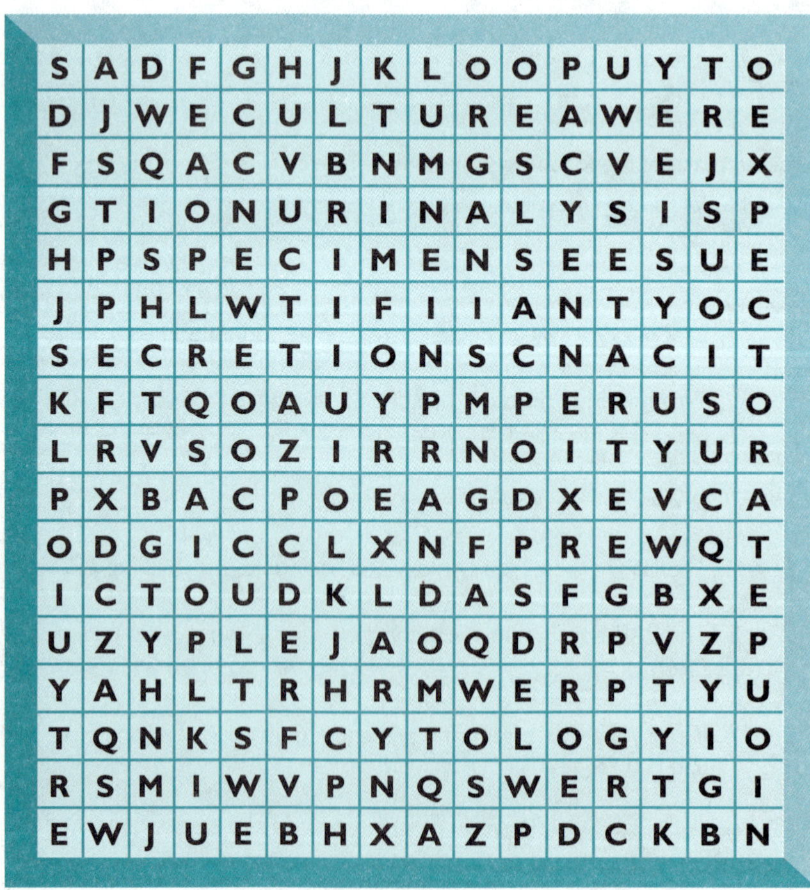

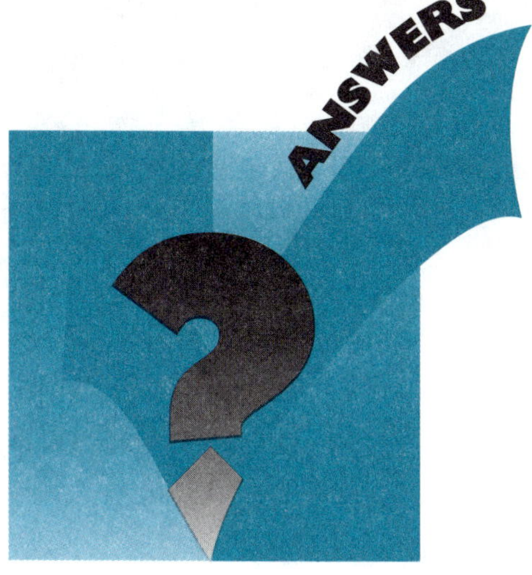

Vocabulary

1. m	4. h	7. f	10. d	13. l
2. e	5. c	8. a	11. o	14. i
3. k	6. j	9. n	12. b	15. g

Student Activities

1. Answers may vary.

2. Answers may vary.

3. Answers may vary. As a suggestion, contact Medical Laboratory Evaluation, a proficiency testing program designed specifically for physician office labs. Dial (800) 338-2746, and press #5.

Discussion Topics

1. Suggestions for obtaining urine specimens from small children:

   a. M. R. Pope, R.N., suggestion in Pediatricks, published by Medical Economics Company, Oradell, NJ 07649, 1974, "To collect frequent urine specimens from an infant, put cotton balls inside the diaper."

   b. As written by Ella M. Woodland, R.N. in Pediatricks published by Medical Economics Company, Oradell, NJ 07649, 1974, "To get a urine specimen from a 7-month old girl, I place a potty in position and then insert a thermometer in the rectum. The baby's reflex "pushing" action produces the specimen without delay."

2. Read "Are Your Gloves Safe?" written by Deney Ward, CMA, POLT, a lab technician in

a community health clinic in Gulfport, Mississippi. The article is printed in the November/December 1993 issue of Professional Medical Assistant, a publication of the American Association of Medical Assistants, pg 6. Additional suggested reading, 55 Federal Register 239.

Review and Rationale

1. Urinalysis can be affected by diet and medications.

2. Urine should not be collected in the bedpan with the stool.

3. Do not throw the tongue depressor or spatula in the wastebasket because it may be contaminated with infectious disease organisms.

4. These foods and drugs may cause a false-positive fecal blood test reading.

5. Helps relax the patient's throat muscle and minimize the gag reflex.

6. This opens up the throat area.

7. To prevent the death of cells.

8. This attaches the microorganisms to the slide.

9. So the movement of the live cells can be viewed under the microscope.

10. In the case of trichomonas organism it must be viewed and identified immediately.

Multiple Choice

1. d	4. e	7. c	10. c	13. a
2. b	5. a	8. d	11. a	14. a
3. c	6. b	9. b	12. b	15. c

True or False

1. T	3. F	5. T	7. T	9. T
2. T	4. F	6. F	8. F	10. F

Word Puzzle

S A D F G H J K L O O P U Y T O
D J W E C U L T U R E A W E R E
F S Q A C V B N M G S C V E J X
G T I O N U R I N A L Y S I S P
H P S P E C I M E N S E E S U E
J P H L W T I F I I A N T Y O C
S E C R E T I O N S C N A C I T
K F T Q O A U Y P M P E R U S O
L R V S O Z I R R N O I T Y U R
P X B A C P O E A G D X E V C A
O D G I C C L X N F P R E W Q T
I C T O U D K L D A S F G B X E
U Z Y P L E J A O Q D R P V Z P
Y A H L T R H R M W E R P T Y U
T Q N K S F C Y T O L O G Y I O
R S M I W V P N Q S W E R T G I
E W J U E B H X A Z P D C K B N

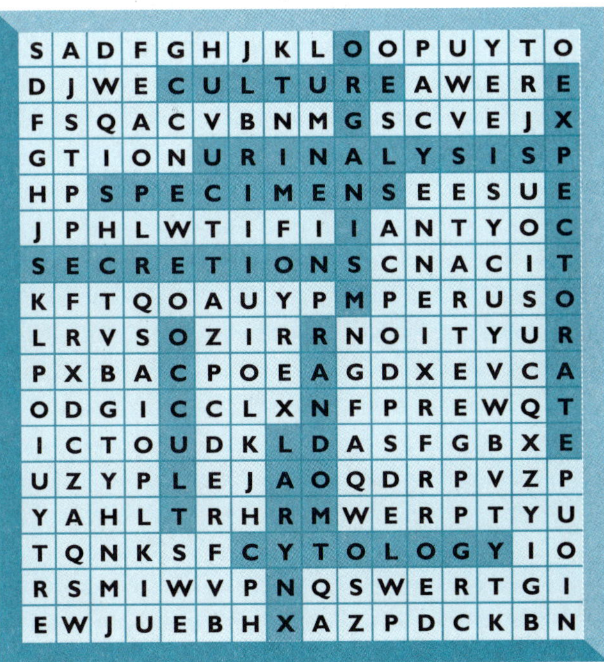

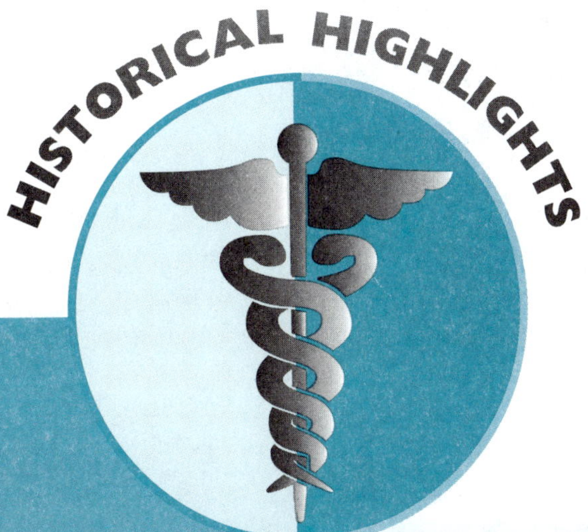

For over 100 centuries drugs have been in use. Substances were thought to possess beneficial effects in the treatment of disease. These "drugs" evolved by way of tradition, and instructions for their use were passed along by word of mouth or reputation. The development of scientific methods for evaluating the effectiveness of drugs has eliminated many of these substances that were used as early drugs. However, there are still remains of the ancient "materia medica" even in modern therapeutics today.

The scientific methods of testing various substances have made it possible to develop new and more effective agents. The resulting new drugs are constantly undergoing change and quite often may be completely outmoded within a year by newer, more potent drugs.

While it is the physician who makes the diagnosis and prescribes the treatment, the pharmacist is the one who is licensed or authorized to dispense drugs. The term apothecary from the Greek apotheke, meaning a storing place, is another name for a druggist or pharmacist. However, the medical assistant has an important responsibility to properly instruct patients in the administration of medications and treatments. Equally important is your observation, reporting, and recording of any undesired effects. It is imperative that you learn as much about drugs as you can and equally important that you understand when, how, and where to use reference materials.

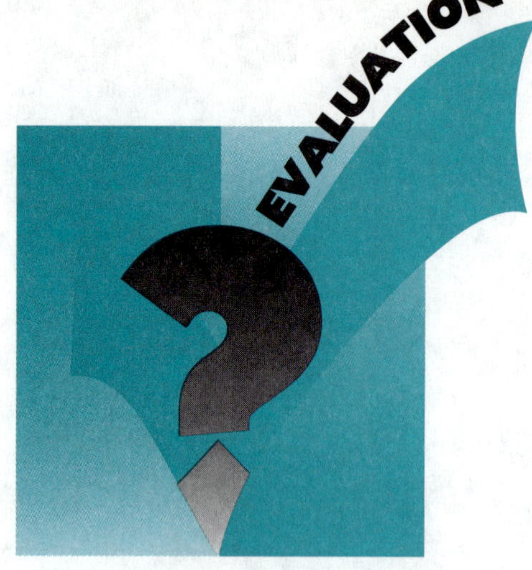

Vocabulary

Write the letter of each term on the line of its matching definition at the right.

a. therapeutic

b. prophylactic

c. diagnostic

d. pill

e. capsules

f. powders

g. suppositories

h. lotions

i. elixirs

j. ointment

k. aerosols

l. injections

m. lumen

n. intramuscular

o. diluents

1. _____ solution of antiseptic or astringent drugs in alcohol or water, applied to the skin as a wash in the treatment of inflammation

2. _____ small containers for drugs which are made of gelatin

3. _____ prevent disease

4. _____ a solution suspended in the form of a mist

5. _____ small pellets of solid drugs molded into the form of spheres

6. _____ treat or cure a disease

7. _____ fluid preparations containing alcohol, syrup and aromatic substances

8. _____ forcing a fluid into a vessel or cavity

9. _____ an agent that dilutes the substances or solution to which it is added

10. _____ solid preparations in which the drug is mixed with a fatty ointment base

11. _____ preparations of drugs mixed with a suppository base such as cacao butter or glycerinated gelatin and molded into special shapes for insertion into the rectum, vagina or urethra

12. _____ medicinal preparations containing finely ground drugs

13. _____ within a muscle

14. _____ space within a tube

15. _____ detect disease

Student Activities

1. The medical assistant should have an understanding of drug standards imposed by various regulatory agencies. Research the following entities:

   a. The Pharmacopeia of the United States

   b. The National Formulary

   c. Federal Drug Administration

   (Your local medical library or pharmacist may be of assistance in your research.)

2. Drugs are derived from many different sources. Compile a list of commonly prescribed and nonprescribed drugs in the following categories:

   a. plants

   b. minerals

   c. animals

   d. synthetics

   e. others

3. A major reference source found in all medical settings is the *Physician's Desk Reference (PDR)*. Using the *PDR*, explore its wealth of information. Then answer the following questions:

   a. Where do you find information about pharmaceutical products produced by a particular manufacturer? What color pages is this information on?

   b. A patient brings in a pill box with several different pills. How do you identify the product? What section of the PDR will be helpful?

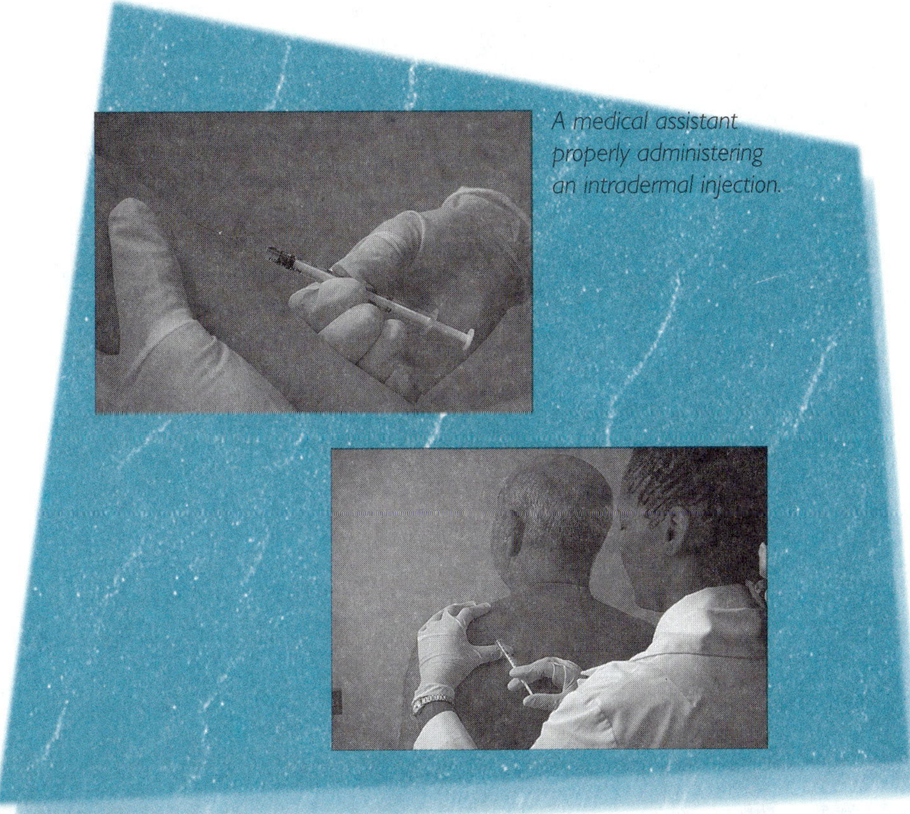

A medical assistant properly administering an intradermal injection.

c. A quick reference section categorizing pharmaceutical products can be found in which colored section of the PDR?

d. If you know the principle ingredient(s) of a drug, in which section can you find the generic and chemical name of the product? What color is this section?

e. An alphabetical sequencing by brand name can be found in which section of the PDR?

Discussion Topics

1. The importance of laws to regulate the importation, manufacture, sale, prescribing, dispensing and possession of narcotic drugs such as opiates, cocaine, and other related compounds including cannabis or marijuana come under federal guidelines. Discuss this in light of current legislation.

2. Before a drug is approved and reaches the market, it must undergo rigorous testing. Quite often drugs for deadly diseases such as cancer and AIDS are available in foreign countries before they are available in the U.S. Discuss the pros and cons of this testing and reasons why drugs must go through this lengthy research.

3. Discuss why drugs are put up in so many forms (for example, pills, caplets, solutions, and spansules).

Review and Rationale

Answer the following questions in the space provided.

1. Why must you always adhere to what are called the five rights of medication administration?

____

____

____

2. Why is it the patient's right and your responsibility to make sure you have followed each of the five rights?

____

____

____

3. Why is a well-lighted area away from distractions and interruptions advisable when administering medications?

____

____

____

4. Why should you ask the patient if there is a known allergy to any medication?

____

____

____

5. Why should a medication be crushed or dissolved and discarded in a sink drain or toilet if the patient refuses it?

____

____

____

6. Why is the medicine bottle cap placed upside down on a flat surface?

____

____

____

7. Why should the plastic graduate cup be held at eye level while pouring?

____

____

____

8. Why should you remain with the patient after administering solid or liquid medication?

____

____

____

9. Why must care be given to locate the correct gluteus medius site when administering an intramuscular injection?

____

____

____

10. Why is the "Z" track injection method an alternate intramuscular injection technique?

____

____

____

11. Why do you rotate injection sites when frequent subcutaneous injections are given?

____

____

____

12. Why do you need to be careful not to touch the needle to the outside of the medication ampule?

____

____

____

13. Why do you push the syringe plunger down, injecting air into the medication vial?

____

____

____

14. Why do you slowly push on the plunger of the filled syringe until a tiny drop of medication comes to the needle tip?

____

____

____

15. Why is the plunger gently pulled back on the syringe, a procedure called aspiration?

____

____

____

Performance Test

In a skills laboratory, a simulation of a job-like environment the medical assistant student must demonstrate skill and knowledge in performing the following procedures without reference to source materials. For these activities, you will need a person to play the role of the patient to demonstrate the correct positioning and locate the correct anatomical site to be used for the injection. An artificial limb may be used for performing the actual injection. Time limits for the performance of each procedure are to be assigned by the instructor.

Administer medication safely and efficiently by accomplishing the following:

1. Administer medication orally
2. Administer medication by intramuscular, subcutaneous, and intradermal injection.

You are expected to perform the above activities with 100% accuracy 90 % of the time (9 out of 10 times).

Performance Checklist

DIRECTIONS: The following checklist will be used to evaluate your performance of each procedure.

Checklist 7-1: Preparing and Administering Drugs (Figure 7-1)

Checklist	S or NA	U	NO	Comment
1. Wash hands.				
2. Maintain Universal Precautions.				
3. Remove medication from storage area and check medication label three times.				
4. Check physician order and medication container for accuracy and drop the tablet into the medication bottle cap.				
5. Transfer the tablet into a medicine cup.				
6. Check the label of the medication and return it to the storage area.				
7. Double check your dosage, bring the written order and the medication to the patient.				
8. Check the patient's identity with the name on the order and remain with the patient until you are certain the medication has been swallowed.				

*S or NA = satisfactory or not applicable; U = unsatisfactory; NO = not observed

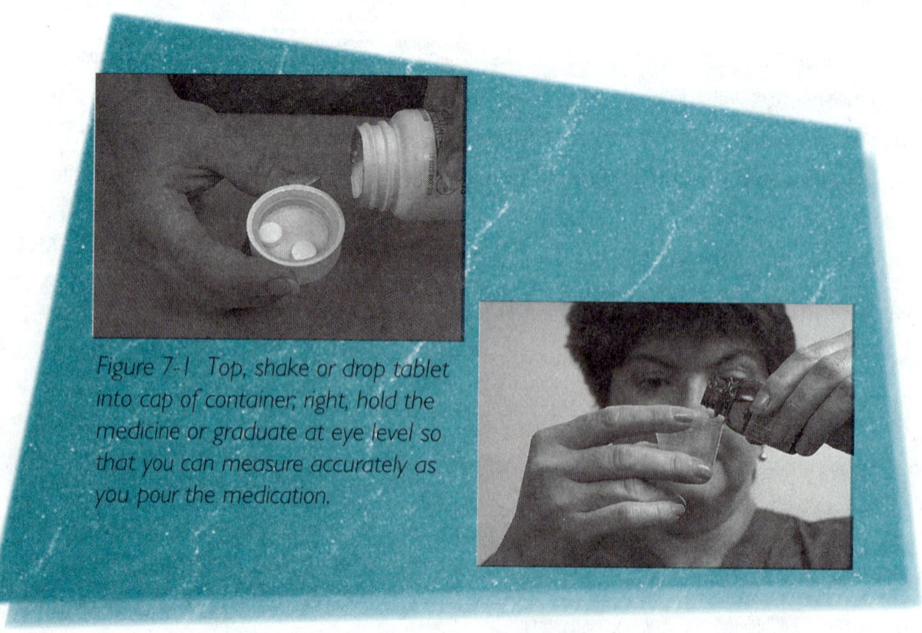

Figure 7-1 *Top, shake or drop tablet into cap of container; right, hold the medicine or graduate at eye level so that you can measure accurately as you pour the medication.*

Checklist 7-2: Administering Drug Injections. Prepare medication for administration by injection using vial.

Checklist	S or NA	U	NO	Comment
1. Wash hands.				
2. Follow Universal Precautions.				
3. Assemble equipment				
4. Prepare syringe and needle for use.				
5. Check the medication label three times as you are preparing the medication for administration.				
6. Calculate correct dosage.				
7. Pull plunger back to acquire a measured amount of air equal to the amount of medication you will withdraw from the vial.				
8. Use an alcohol sponge to cleanse vial.				
9. Remove needle cover, insert the needle through the cleansed, rubber stopper of vial and keep the inserted needle above the solution.				
10. Push the syringe plunger down, injecting the air into the vial.				
11. Invert the vial and the syringe, bringing them to eye level.				
12. Draw the plunger back gently.				
13. Draw up the correct amount of medication and remove the needle from the vial, replacing the needle cover.				
14. Place the filled syringe with the covered needle and the alcohol sponges on a clean, small tray.				
15. Check the label on the vial with the physician's order and replace or discard the medication vial.				

*S or NA = satisfactory or not applicable; U = unsatisfactory; NO = not observed

Checklist 7-3: Intramuscular Injections. Administer medication by intramuscular injection using a disposable plastic syringe into the gluteus medius muscle.

Checklist	S or NA	U	NO	Comment
1. Wash hands.				
2. Follow Universal Precautions.				
3. Assemble equipment.				
4. Identify the patient and explain the procedure.				
5. Select the injection site and position the patient.				
6. Cleanse injection site.				
7. Remove needle cover and expel the air.				
8. With a quick, dart-like thrust, insert the needle at a 90 degree angle to about $3/4$ the needle length.				
9. Gently pull back on the plunger; if no blood is aspirated, inject the medication.				
10. Apply pressure at the site with the alcohol sponge and quickly remove the needle.				
11. Place the syringe and needle on the tray.				
12. Massage the injection site with the sponge.				
13. Assist patient to a safe and comfortable position and observe for any unusual reactions.				
14. Inform patient if he/she is free to leave.				
15. Dispose of the needle and syringe in a designated used sharps container.				
16. Wash your hands.				
17. Record the entire procedure on the patient's chart.				

*S or NA = satisfactory or not applicable; U = unsatisfactory; NO = not observed

Checklist 7-4: Subcutaneous Injections. (See Figure 7-3) Administer medication by subcutaneous injection using a disposable plastic syringe into the outer surface of the upper arm.

Checklist	S or NA	U	NO	Comment
1. Wash hands.				
2. Follow Universal Precautions.				
3. Assemble equipment.				
4. Identify the patient and explain the procedure.				
5. Put on gloves.				
6. Cleanse injection site with alcohol sponge.				
7. Slowly push on the plunger to expel the air from the syringe.				
8. Locate the injection site and position the patient.				
9. Remove needle cover and expel air.				
10. Inject the medication by holding the needle and syringe at a 45 degree angle.				
11. Pull back on plunger; inject medication slowly.				
12. Apply pressure with an alcohol sponge to the injection site and remove needle.				
13. Massage injection site and observe for any patient reactions.				
14. Assure patient safety and comfort; provide any further instructions.				
15. Dispose of needle and syringe in a designated used sharps container.				
16. Wash your hands.				
17. Record the entire procedure on the patient's chart.				

*S or NA = satisfactory or not applicable; U = unsatisfactory; NO = not observed

Checklist 7-5: Intradermal Injections. Administer medication by intradermal injection using a disposable plastic syringe into the inner surface of the forearm.

Checklist	S or NA	U	NO	Comment
1. Wash hands.				
2. Follow Universal Precautions.				
3. Assemble equipment.				
4. Prepare syringe and needle for use.				
5. Identify the patient and explain the procedure.				
6. Select the injection site and position the patient.				
7. Put on gloves.				
8. Cleanse injection site with alcohol sponge.				
9. Slowly push on the plunger to expel the air from the syringe.				
10. Administer the intradermal injection by holding the needle bevel side up and the syringe at a 10 to 15 degree angle.				
11. Inject the medication slowly.				
12. Apply pressure at the site with the alcohol sponge and quickly remove the needle.				
13. Place the syringe and needle on the tray.				
14. Massage the injection site with the sponge.				
15. Assist patient to a safe and comfortable position and observe for any unusual reactions.				
16. Inform patient if he/she is free to leave.				
17. Dispose of the needle and syringe in a designated used sharps container.				
18. Wash your hands.				
19. Record the entire procedure on the patient's chart.				

*S or NA = satisfactory or not applicable; U = unsatisfactory; NO = not observed

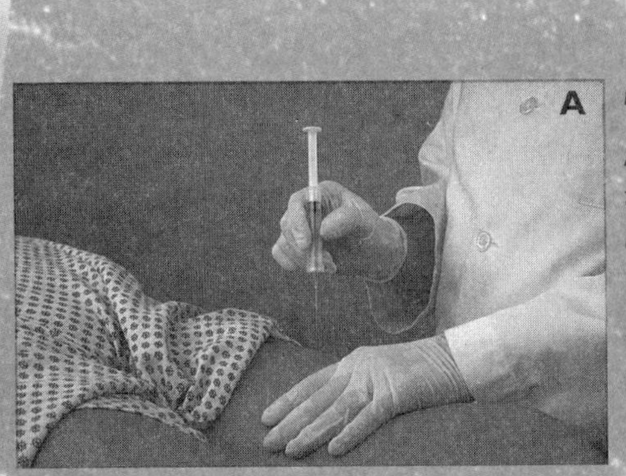

Figure 7-2

A. *Giving intramuscular injections. Hold syringe and needle in pencil or dartlike grip;*

B. *Insert at 90-degree angle with a quick thrust. Do note hit skin with hub of needle.*

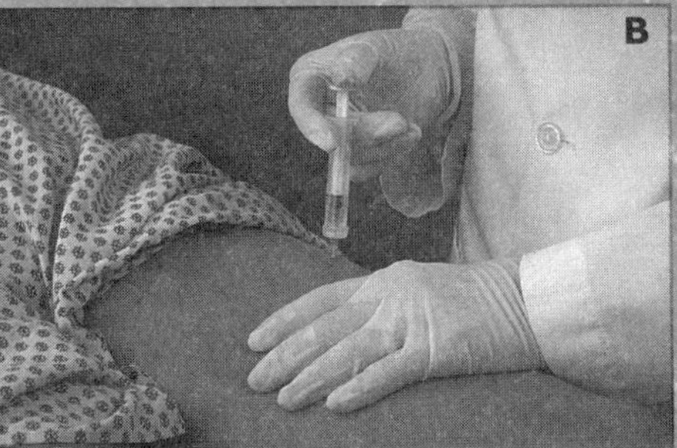

Figure 7-3 Technique for administering a subcutaneous injection. Insert needle at a 45-degree angle.

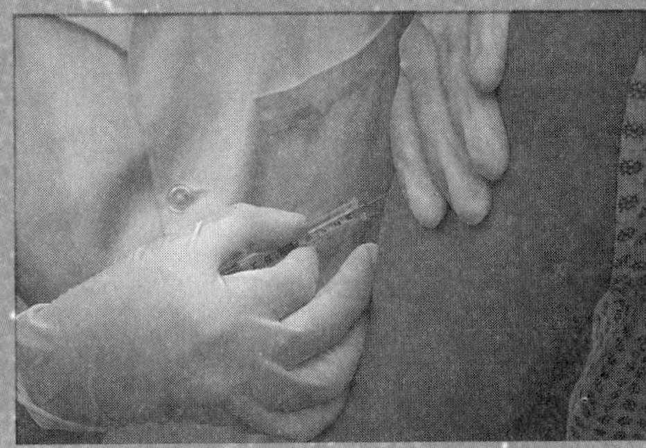

Figure 7-4 Angles of insertion for parenteral injections.

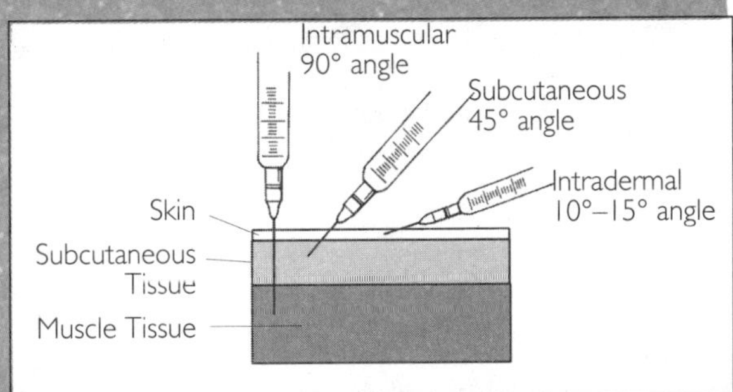

Multiple Choice

From the options listed under each question or statement, select the correct answer or answers. Write the corresponding letter or letters in the answer space.

1. Pharmacology is the: _______
   a. science that deals with the study of drugs.
   b. science that deals with the origin of drugs.
   c. science that deals with the study of drug characteristics, uses, and actions.
   d. all of the above.

2. All but one of the following are solid state drugs: _______
   a. spansules
   b. caplets
   c. suppositories
   d. elixirs

3. The most commonly used needle size ranges from: _______
   a. $1/4$ inch to 2 inches
   b. $1/2$ inch to $5/8$ inch
   c. $3/8$ inch to $1\,1/2$ inches
   d. none of the above

4. The TB syringe uses a: _______
   a. 20 or 21 gauge, $5/8$ inch needle
   b. 21 or 22 gauge, $1\,1/2$ inch needle
   c. 26 or 27 gauge, $3/8$ or $1/2$ inch needle
   d. any of the above

5. The most common site for an intradermal injection is the: _______
   a. inner surface of the forearm about 4 inches below the elbow
   b. the outer surface of the upper arm
   c. upper $2/3$ of the back
   d. lateral aspect to the thigh

6. Subcutaneous injections are given at a _______ degree angle:
   a. 10–15
   b. 45
   c. 90
   d. 75

7. Single use medications are supplied in: _________
   a. prefilled syringes or cartridges
   b. glass ampules
   c. vials
   d. all of the above

8. Too much air pressure in the vial will cause the solution in the syringe to: _________
   a. plug the needle
   b. create a vacuum
   c. make it difficult to draw up an accurate dosage
   d. cause air bubbles to develop in the syringe

9. Intradermal injections are administered by holding the needle and the syringe at a
   _____________degree angle:
   a. 10–15
   b. 45
   c. 74
   d. 90

10. Liquid state medications include: _________
   a. spansules
   b. emulsions
   c. caplets
   d. suppositories

Brief Answer

Answer each question or complete the statement in the space provided.

1. List the five rights of medication administration.

   a. ____

   b. ____

   c. ____

   d. ____

   e. ____

2. Before administering any drug, there are general supplies and procedures which you
must follow. First, you will need a ________________________, the correct
________________________ to be administered, a pen and paper and the patient's
________________.

3. Understand as much as you can about the drug you are giving. Know how the drug is
usually ________________, what a patient's typical reaction will be, what the drug
____________, and what the normal ________________ is.

4. Maintain Universal Precautions when administering oral drugs in ___________________ form.

5. Injections are administered when a _______________ response to a drug is desired.

True or False

Determine whether each of the following statements is true or false. Check the box marked T or F at the left of the statement.

T F

☐ ☐ 1. Inaccuracy in any of the medication administration procedures can lead to serious drug reactions within the patient and possibly even death.

☐ ☐ 2. A slight deviation from the prescribed dosage is acceptable.

☐ ☐ 3. Drugs are supplied only in solid state and must be dissolved into liquid for injected or oral administration.

☐ ☐ 4. If a patient refuses a tablet, crush it and discard it in the trash receptacle.

☐ ☐ 5. Do not leave medication unattended on medcarts or counters.

☐ ☐ 6. Shake any medication which is in the form of an emulsion or suppository.

☐ ☐ 7. Remove the medicine bottle cap and place it rightside up on a flat surface so that the sterile inside of the cap is not contaminated.

☐ ☐ 8. Check the medication label prior to returning it to the storage area.

☐ ☐ 9. Check all medication labels three times during preparation and administration procedures.

☐ ☐ 10. Use a longer, thinner needle on children or thin patients.

Word Puzzle

Circle the following medical terms related to pharmacology and drug administration.

injections	lumen	ointment
diagnostic	suppositories	prophylactic
intramuscular	lotions	capsules
spansules	elixirs	aerosols

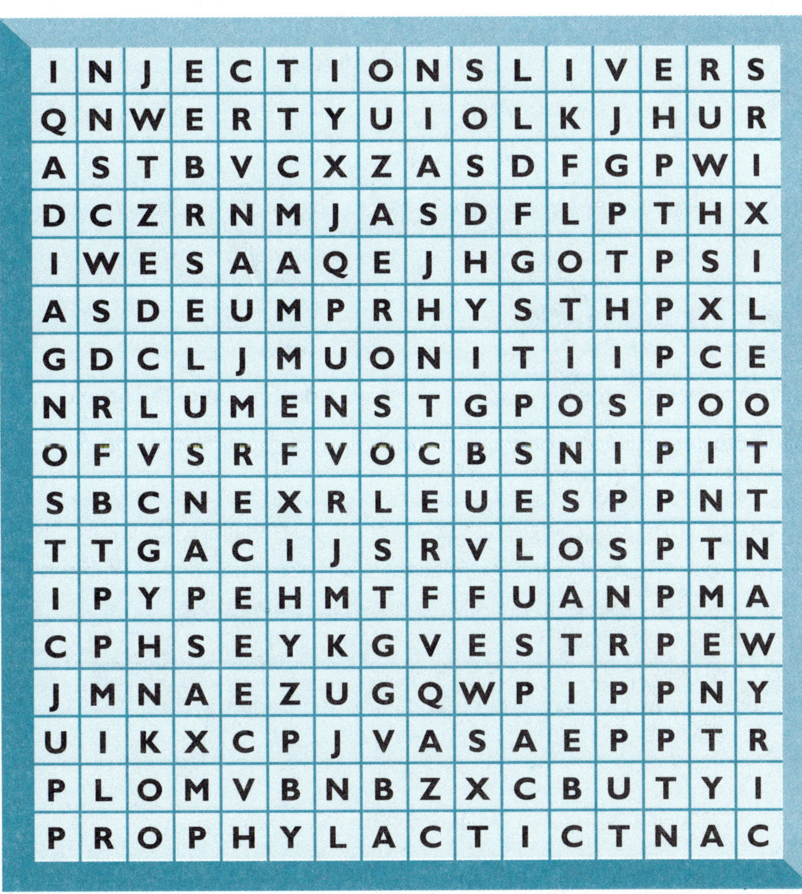

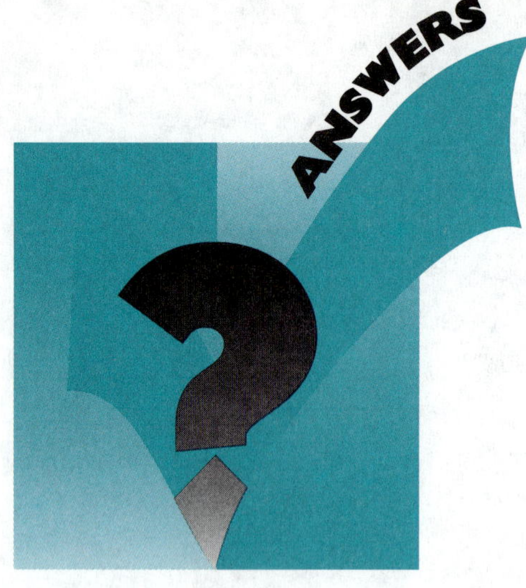

Vocabulary

1. h	4. k	7. i	10. j	13. n
2. e	5. d	8. l	11. g	14. m
3. b	6. a	9. o	12. f	15. c

Student Activities

1. a. The Pharmacopeia of the United States contains a description of the source, appearance, properties, standards of purity and similar information of the most important and most frequently used drugs.

    b. The National Formulary contains a description of drugs that are not sufficiently important to be included in the Pharmacopeia and also a description of important standard mixtures of drugs frequently employed in prescriptions.

    c. Federal Drug Administration is the enforcement agency for the standards of purity and potency set by the Pharmacopeia and National Formulary.

2. Answers may vary.

3. a. Section 1: Manufacturers' Index (white pages)

    b. Start by comparing the pills with the full-color reproductions of tablets, caplets, and capsules selected for inclusion by participating manufacturers of drugs in the Product Identification Section.

    c. Section 3: Product Category Index (green pages)

    d. Section 4: Generic and Chemical Name Index (yellow pages)

    e. Section 2: Product Name Index (pink pages)

Discussion Topics

1. Answers may vary.

2. Answers may vary; however, the activity might include investigation into the type of action the drug produces in an animal, such as anesthesia, relief of pain, relaxation of smooth muscles, which might be of value in the treatment of disease in humans. The drug might show if it possesses any other effects which might be dangerous in humans.

Answers may vary in discussion of the pros and cons; for example, animal testing.

3. Answers may vary.

Review and Rationale

1. You must be sure that you are administering the right drug; at the right dose; by the right route for administration; at the right time; to the right patient.

2. Inaccuracy in any of the medication administration procedures can lead to serious drug reactions within the patient and possibly even death.

3. To assure that you prepare the right drug at the right dose, remain in a well-lighted area away from distractions and interruptions.

4. If there is a possibility that the patient is allergic to a prescribed drug, the physician must be notified so a substitute can be found.

5. Refused medication must be properly discarded because once it has been removed from its sterile container, it is considered contaminated.

6. By placing the medicine bottle cap upside down on a flat surface, its cap will remain sterile and not become contaminated.

7. To assure greater accuracy, hold the medicine and plastic graduate cup at eye level while pouring.

8. Remain with the patient until you are certain that the solid or liquid has been swallowed.

9. Take care to locate the correct gluteus medium site to avoid hitting the sciatic nerve or the superior gluteal artery.

10. The "Z" pattern tract keeps medication deep in the muscle and prevents seepage through the skin.

11. Rotate injection sites to prevent damage to the tissue, excessive pain, and possible disfigurement.

12. Touching the needle to the outside of the medication ampule would contaminate the sterile needle and another one would need to be obtained.

13. Too much air pressure in the vial will force the solution into the syringe, making it difficult to draw up an accurate dosage so it is important not to inject more air than is required.

14. Slowly pushing on the plunger until a tiny drop of medication comes to the needle tip expels the air from the syringe, and ensures that the needle is not plugged.

15. This is done to determine if the needle entered a blood vessel in which case the needle must be withdrawn, changed, and the injection begun again using a new site.

Multiple Choice

1. d	3. a	5. a	7. d	9. a
2. d	4. c	6. b	8. c	10. b

Brief Answer

1. a. right drug
   b. right dose
   c. right route
   d. right time
   e. right patient

2. physician's accurately written medication order, dosage of drug, chart

3. administered, trents, dosage

4. tablet

5. rapid

True or False

1. T	3. F	5. T	7. F	9. T
2. F	4. F	6. F	8. T	10. F

Word Puzzle

I N J E C T I O N S L I V E R S
Q N W E R T Y U I O L K J H U R
A S T B V C X Z A S D F G P W I
D C Z R N M J A S D F L P T H X
I W E S A A Q E J H G O T P S I
A S D E U M P R H Y S T H P X L
G D C L J M U O N I T I I P C E
N R L U M E N S T G P O S P O O
O F V S R F V O C B S N I P I T
S B C N E X R L E U E S P P N T
T T G A C I J S R V L O S P T N
I P Y P E H M T F F U A N P M A
C P H S E Y K G V E S T R P E W
J M N A E Z U G Q W P I P P N Y
U I K X C P J V A S A E P P T R
P L O M V B N B Z X C B U T Y I
P R O P H Y L A C T I C T N A C

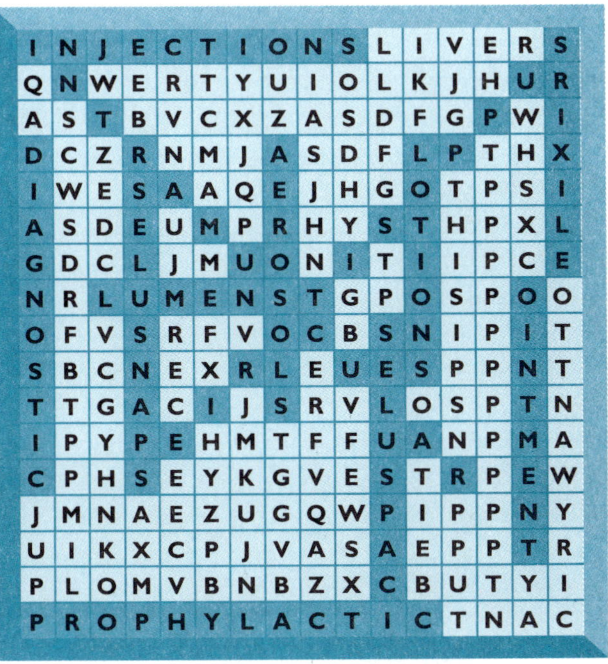

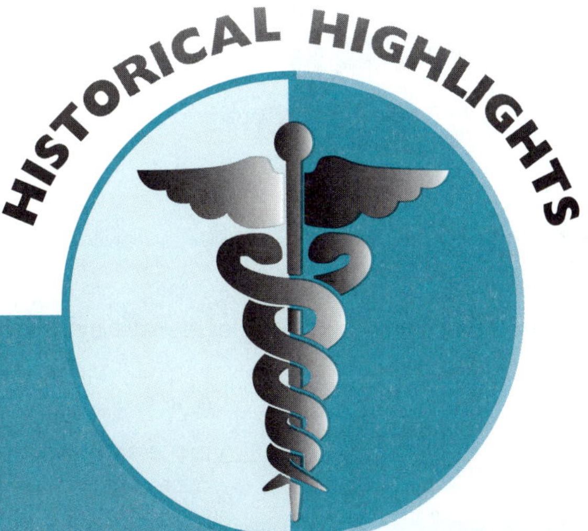

Tuberculosis *(TB)* is a disease caused by bacilli that are rod-shaped. *TB* is also known as *consumption* and has been recognized as a disease from the earliest times of recorded history. From 460 to 375 B.C. Hippocrates, the father of medicine, called the disease *phthisis,* meaning affected with *pulmonary* tuberculosis. While TB commonly affects the respiratory system, other parts of the body such as *gastrointestinal* and *genitourinary* tracts, skeletal and nervous system may also become infected. In 980 A.D., Haly Abbas of Baghdad recognized the infectious nature of phthisis. This theory was again pursued in the 1700s. After the middle of the nineteenth century, it was proven by means of *inoculation* techniques that tuberculosis is really an infectious *malady.* It was not until the late 1880's when Koch made an announcement of the discovery of the *tubercle bacillus,* or germ or bacteria.

Early diagnosis and effective treatment of tuberculosis is responsible for the decline of this once prevalent disease. TB affected people regardless of their social or economic status. In recent years, however, TB has begun to creep back into our society. The medical assistant should be aware of this more current outbreak of tuberculosis and constantly strive to be alert to new strains of the disease and methods of detection.

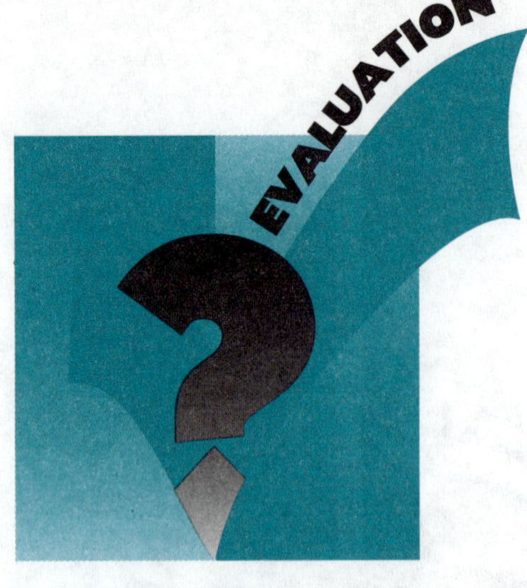

Vocabulary

Write the letter of each term on the line of its matching definition at the right.

a. Tine test

b. tuberculosis

c. volar

d. Charles Mantoux

e. induration

f. instillations

g. irrigations

h. otoscope

i. OD

j. OS

k. OU

l. TB

m. conjunctiva

n. secretions

o. saline

p. boric acid

1. _____ right eye

2. _____ process whereby cells of glandular organs produce certain materials from the blood

3. _____ dropping of fluid or ointment into a body cavity

4. _____ inside surface of forearm

5. _____ mucous membrane that lines eyelids and is reflected onto eyeball

6. _____ an infectious disease caused by the tubercle bacillus

7. _____ both eyes

8. _____ test that screen patients for the presence of tuberculosis

9. _____ flushing or washing of an area with a stream of fluid

10. _____ abbreviation for disease described in #6 above

11. _____ hardened tissue

12. _____ left eye

13. _____ containing salt

14. _____ instrument to examine the ear

15. _____ French physician

16. _____ a white, odorless powder or crystalline substance used as a buffer and formerly employed as a topical antiseptic and eye wash

Student Activities

1. Visit your community hospital library or other medical research center and investigate the following questions:

   a. What are the reasons behind the recent increase in the number of reported tuberculosis cases?

   b. What role does the state play in the payment, treatment, and assurance of patient compliance in the treatment of tuberculosis?

2. Often children insert small objects into their ears. The use of an otoscope is required, but many children are frightened of instruments and refuse to cooperate during the examination. Here is a story devised by Dennis Fitzgerald, M.D. to help during examination of the child whom he suspects has a foreign body lodged in his ear.

   Where's the Birdie? When a small child refuses to sit still for an ear examination, try entering his world of make-believe with this trick: Tell him you think you hear a bird chirping in one of his ears, and that you are going to try to find it with your bird-finder (otoscope). After a search of both ears fails to turn up the bird, the child will no longer be frightened of the otoscope and will be more cooperative during the examination.

What other "tricks" can be used to gain the confidence and cooperation of young patients who must undergo ear instillations and irrigations?

3. Pharmaceuticals are prescribed by the physician using metric doses. When tablets, capsules and pills are prescribed in the metric system, the pharmacist may dispense the corresponding approximate equivalent in the apothecary system or vice versa. Use a conversion table to complete the following exercise:

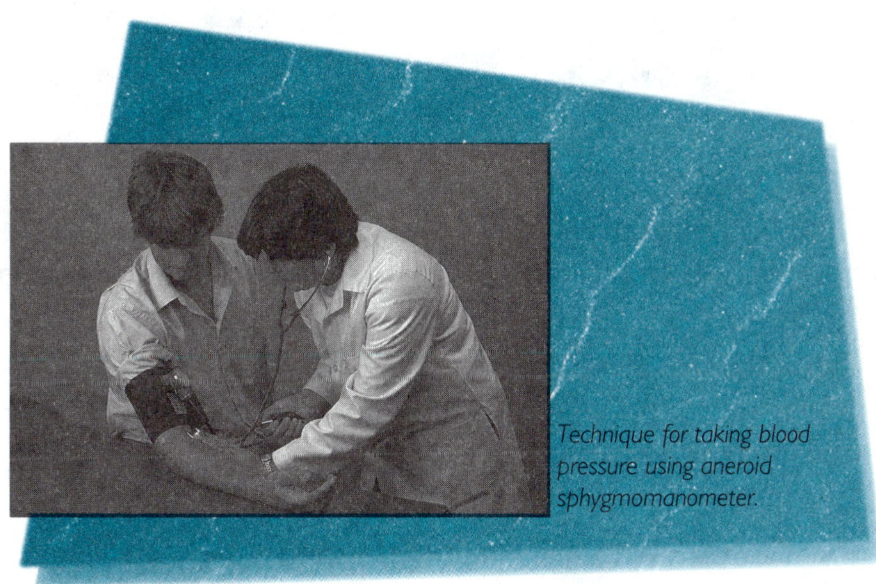

Technique for taking blood pressure using aneroid sphygmomanometer.

	LIQUID MEASURE		WEIGHT	
Metric		Approximate Apothecary Equivalents	Metric	Approximate Apothecary Equivalents
250 mL			30 grams	
30 mL			3 g	
	30 grains ($^1/_2$ dram)			$^1/_{10}$ grain
1000 mL				$^1/_{40}$ grain
	3$^1/_2$ fluid ounces			22 grains

4. Using the most recent edition of the *Physician's Desk Reference* or other guide to prescription drugs, choose one drug and answer the following questions:

    a. What are several brand names for this drug.

    b. Why is this drug prescribed?

    c. What important side effects may occur?

    d. When should this drug be discontinued?

    e. Are there any special warnings about this medication?

    f. Are there any possible food or drug interactions when taking this medication?

    g. What is the recommended dosage?

    h. What constitutes overdosage?

    i. What special instructions or warnings apply if the patient is pregnant or breast-feeding?

Discussion Topics

1. Health care workers are tested yearly for the presence of a positive tuberculin test. Contact your community hospital and inquire as to the type of test performed. If the PPD (purified protein derivative) intradermal injection is used in place of the Tine test, why is it the preferred test? What are the consequences to the community of a health care worker who is found to have a positive test result? …to the patient? …to his/her family?

2. For better patient compliance, your ability to give instructions about medications and treatment is crucial. Role playing and practice sessions related to instructing patients will be valuable to you. Set up role playing with a partner, taking turns being the medical assistant and the patient. The patient can portray various age categories and disabilities to make the

activity more realistic. For example: portray a child, adolescent, young adult, middle aged and elderly patient; vary the disabilities represented (hearing, visual, language and being wheelchair bound). Ask other classmates to critique the instruction session.

Review and Rationale

Answer the following questions in the space provided.

1. When administering the tine unit, why grasp the upper third of the patient's forearm on the posterior side?

____

____

____

2. Following puncture of the skin with the tine disc, why must it be held in place for one second?

____

____

____

3. Why is it important to ask the patient if he/she has had drainage from the ear or any complications from previous irrigations?

____

____

____

4. Why should the patient be instructed to sit with the head tilted slightly toward the affected side when irrigating the ear?

____

____

____

5. When placing the tip of the syringe at the opening of the ear, why should the tip be pointed upward and toward the back of the canal?

____

____

____

6. What should you do if the patient exhibits signs of discomfort or dizziness when irrigating the ear?

____

____

____

7. After instilling eye drops, why should the patient be instructed to close the eyelid and move the eye?

____

____

____

8. When instilling eye ointment, why must care be taken not to touch the eyelid?

____

____

____

9. As a medical assistant, why is it your responsibility to always follow the five rights of medication administration?

____

____

____

10. When working with the eyes and ears, why must they be treated gently?

____

____

____

Performance Test

In a skills laboratory, a simulation of a job-like environment, the medical student must demonstrate knowledge and skill in performing the following procedures without reference to source materials. Time limits for the performance of each procedure are to be assigned by the instructor.

1. Tine Tuberculin Test
2. Ear instillation
3. Ear irrigation
4. Eye instillation
5. Eye irrigation

You are expected to perform the above activities with 100% accuracy 90% of the time (9 out of 10 times).

Performance Checklist

DIRECTIONS: The following checklist will be used to evaluate your performance of each procedure.

Checklist 8-1: Tine Tuberculin Test (Figure 8-1)

Checklist	S or NA	U	NO	Comment
1. Wash your hands.				
2. Assemble supplies.				
3. Identify patient and explain procedure.				
4. Put on gloves.				
5. Position, support, and expose patient's forearm.				
6. Cleanse skin.				
7. Remove protective cap on tine unit.				
8. Grasp forearm; with your dominant hand, puncture the skin with the tine unit; hold for one second.				
9. Discard tine unit in designated used sharps container.				
10. Instruct patient.				
11. Wash hands.				
12. Record information on patient's medical record.				
Upon return of patient for examination:				
13. Inspect injection site.				
14. Record the time and results on the patient's medical record.				

*S or NA = satisfactory or not applicable; U = unsatisfactory; NO = not observed

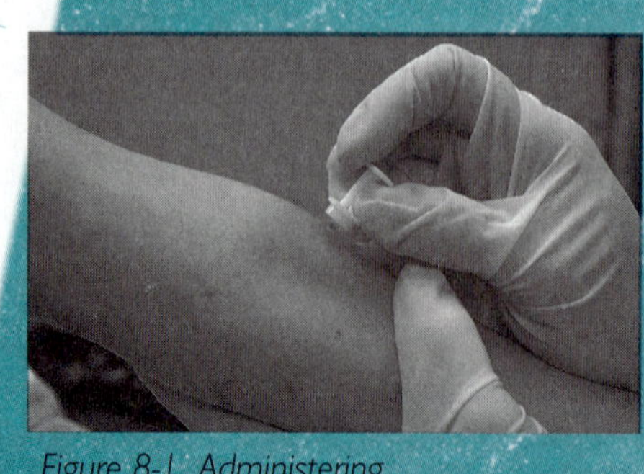

Figure 8-1 *Administering the tine tuberculin test.*

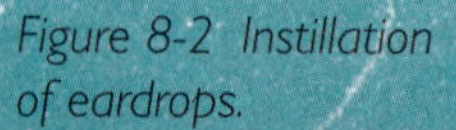

Figure 8-2 *Instillation of eardrops.*

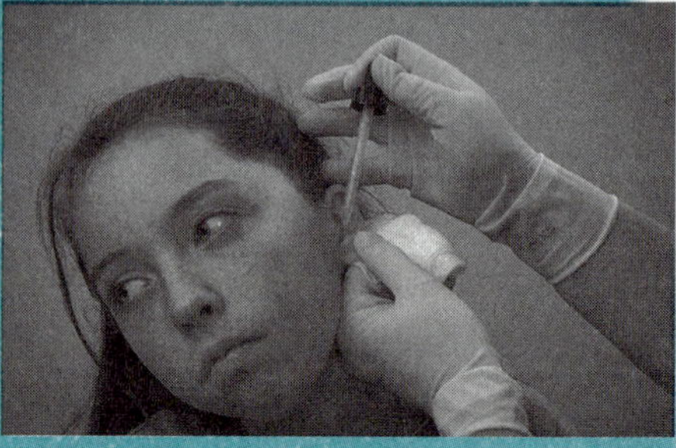

Checklist 8-2: Ear Instillation (See Figure 8-2)

Checklist	S or NA	U	NO	Comment
1. Check medication order and correct ear.				
2. Wash hands.				
3. Assemble supplies.				
4. Read medication label three times.				
5. Check which ear requires treatment.				
6. Identify patient; explain nature and purpose of the procedure.				
7. Position patient in a side-lying or in a sitting position.				
8. Put on gloves.				
9. Instruct patient to tilt head toward the unaffected side.				
10. Stand at the patient's head.				
11. Draw medication into the dropper and examine dropper for any defects.				
12. Straighten patient's external ear canal.				
13. Place the tip of the dropper inside the external ear canal and instill the medication.				
14. Instruct patient to keep the head tilted or remain lying on the unaffected side for a few minutes.				
15. If ordered, place a cotton ball over the opening of the ear.				
16. Discard unused medication before replacing the dropper into the bottle.				
17. Attend to the patient; provide further instructions when required.				
18. Remove and dispose of gloves in appropriate container.				
19. Replace supplies.				
20. Wash your hands.				
21. Record procedure and results in the patient's record.				

*S or NA = satisfactory or not applicable; U = unsatisfactory; NO = not observed

Video 8: Pharmacology & Drug Administration II

Checklist 8-3: Ear Irrigation (See Figure 8-3)

Checklist	S or NA	U	NO	Comment
1. Check medication order and correct ear.				
2. Wash hands.				
3. Assemble supplies.				
4. Check solution label three times; warm the solution.				
5. Identify the patient; explain the nature and purpose of the procedure.				
6. Put on gloves.				
7. Sit the patient with head tilted slightly toward the affected side.				
8. Drape patient's shoulder.				
9. Have patient hold the basin under the ear and against the neck.				
10. Cleanse outer ear and external auditory canal.				
11. Test temperature of the solution.				
12. Fill the syringe with irrigation solution and expel any air present.				
13. Straighten patient's ear canal.				
14. Place tip of the syringe at the opening; slowly and gently direct a steady stream of solution against the roof of the canal.				
15. Observe the patient for signs of discomfort or dizziness.				
16. Continue until desired results are obtained.				
17. Dry external ear with a cotton ball.				
18. Have patient maintain the position for a few minutes.				
19. Remove soiled drapes; provide for patient's safety and comfort; provide further instructions as necessary.				
20. Return supplies.				
21. Remove and discard gloves in appropriate container.				
22. Wash your hands.				
23. Record the procedure in the patient's medical record.				

*S or NA = satisfactory or not applicable; U = unsatisfactory; NO = not observed

Checklist 8-4: Eye Instillation (See Figure 8-4)

Checklist	S or NA	U	NO	Comment
1. Check the medication order and for the correct eye.				
2. Wash hands.				
3. Assemble supplies.				
4. Check medication label three times.				
5. Identify the patient; explain the procedure and purpose.				
6. Put on gloves.				
7. Have patient sit with head tilted slightly backward.				
8. Stand at the patient's head.				
9. Draw medication, and examine dropper for any defects.				
10. With fingers over a tissue, draw the lower lid down gently and have the patient look up.				
11. Hold the dropper parallel to the eye; instill the correct amount of medication into the middle of the conjunctival sac of the lower lid. (To instill ointment, gently squeeze a thin strip of ointment from the tube along the lower lid. Do not touch the eye or the lid.)				
12. Instruct patient to close, but not squeeze eyelid and move the eye.				
13. Wipe off excess medication that flows onto the eye or cheek.				
14. Discard unused solution before replacing the dropper into the bottle. Avoid contamination of the dropper.				
15. Assure safety and comfort of patient; provide further instructions.				
16. Replace supplies.				
17. Remove and discard gloves.				
18. Wash your hands.				
19. Record the procedure on the patient's medical record.				

*S or NA = satisfactory or not applicable; U = unsatisfactory; NO = not observed

Checklist 8-5: Eye Irrigation

Checklist	S or NA	U	NO	Comment
1. Check the medication order and review which eye is to be treated.				
2. Wash hands.				
3. Assemble supplies.				
4. Check the label of the solution three times.				
5. Identify patient; explain the nature and purpose of the procedure. Instruct the patient not to squeeze the eyelids during the treatment.				
6. Place patient in sitting or lying position with the head tilted backward and toward the side being treated.				
7. Place the kidney basin on top of the towel, in a position to receive excess eye irrigation solution.				
8. Stand in front of or to the side of the patient.				
9. Cleanse the eyelid.				
10. Fill the dropper or syringe with solution. Gently draw the lower lid down; instruct the patient to look up and not to squeeze the eyelids.				
11. Squeeze the solution into the eye, allowing it to flow away from the nose.				
12. Do not allow the dropper or syringe to touch the eye or eyelid.				
13. Continue the procedure until the desired results occur or the prescribed amount of solution is used.				
14. Gently dry the eye and cheek with cotton balls; discard cotton balls in a designated container.				
15. Provide for patient's safety and comfort and furnish further instructions as necessary.				
16. Observe the drainage in the basin.				
17. Discard the drainage and soiled disposable items; return reusable supplies to the designated area.				
18. Wash hands.				
19. Record the procedure on the patient's medical record.				

*S or NA = satisfactory or not applicable; U = unsatisfactory; NO = not observed

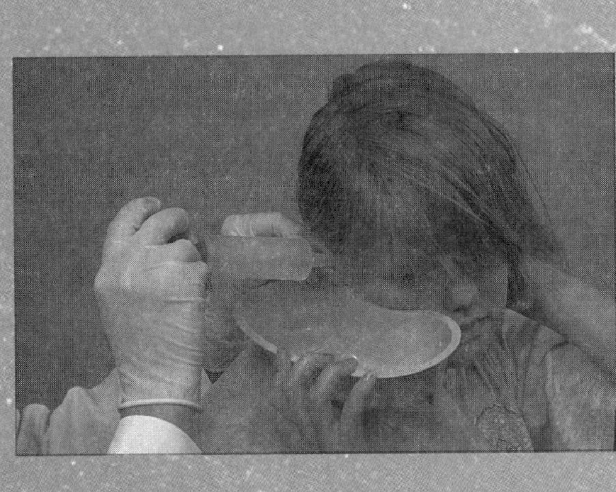

Figure 8-3 Ear irrigation. Have patient hold kidney or ear basin under ear and against the neck. Head should be tilted toward the affected side. Pull earlobe up and backward. Place tip of syringe in ear pointing up and back, and gently direct a steady slow stream of solution against the roof of the ear canal.

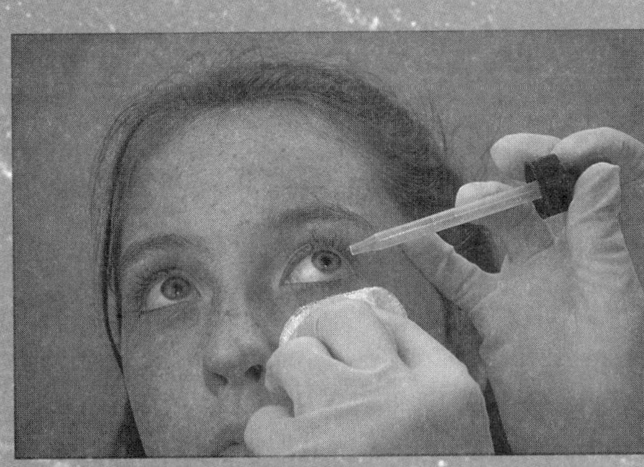

Figure 8-4 Instilling eyedrops. Hold eyedropper parallel to eye to avoid injury to eye of patient.

Multiple Choice

From the option listed under each question or statement, select the correct answer or answers. Write the corresponding letter or letters in the answer space.

1. A test performed using a stainless steel disc with four prongs attached to the handle is called: _______
   a. PPD test
   b. TB test
   c. Tine Tuberculin test
   d. Mantoux test

2. Ear instillations are performed to: _______
   a. soften ear wax
   b. instill medication
   c. help combat inner ear infections
   d. all of the above

3. If a patient has a positive tine test, all of the following except one may be ordered by the physician: _______
   a. chest x-ray
   b. laboratory examination of sputum
   c. PPD test
   d. Factor VIII Assay

4. The patient should be instructed to return for inspection of the induration following the tine test in: _______
   a. 12-24 hours
   b. 24-36 hours
   c. 36-48 hours
   d. 48-72 hours

5. The resulting induration following a tine test of 2-4 mm suggests: _______
   a. doubtful reaction
   b. negative reaction
   c. positive reaction
   d. questionable reaction requiring repeat testing

6. Firmly grasping the patient's forearm on the under side while administering the tine test: _______
   a. stabilizes the patient's arm
   b. allows you to tightly stretch the skin
   c. a and b
   d. none of the above

7. Eye medications may be in the form of: ________
   a. liquid
   b. liquid suspension
   c. sterile ointment
   d. ointment

8. Puncture the skin with the prongs of the tine unit and hold in place for: ________
   a. 1 second
   b. 2 seconds
   c. 3 seconds
   d. 4 seconds

9. Eye medication instillations are performed to: ________
   a. dilate or constrict the pupil of the eye
   b. relieve eye pain and inflammation
   c. anesthetize the eye
   d. stimulate circulation
   e. all of the above

10. The preferred test site for the tine test is: ________
    a. lateral portion of the upper arm
    b. upper third of the posterior of the patient's forearm
    c. volar surface of the upper 1/3 of the forearm
    d. any of the above

True or False

Determine whether each of the following statements is true or false. Check the box marked T or F at the left of the statement.

T F

1. Straighten the external auditory canal of an adult patient by gently pulling the top of the earlobe upward and backward.

2. Explain to the patient that medication may feel cool and flinching or squeezing the eye when it is instilled should be avoided.

3. Replace any unused solution from the dropper into the bottle.

4. Eye irrigations are performed to relieve inflammation of the conjunctiva.

5. Always place a cotton ball over the opening of the ear following instillation of medication.

T   F

☐   ☐   6. Visually examine the eye with an otoscope before performing irrigation.

☐   ☐   7. To dislodge wax or foreign bodies from the external auditory canal, use a cotton-tipped applicator.

☐   ☐   8. If the patient is restless or jerky, be sure to support the head well.

☐   ☐   9. Straighten the external auditory canal of a child by gently pulling the top of the earlobe upward and backward.

☐   ☐   10. Irrigation of the ear is done to relieve inflammation of the ear.

Word Puzzle

Circle the following medical terms related to pharmacy and drug administration.

boric acid	otoscope	Charles Mantoux
saline	irrigations	volar
secretions	instillations	tuberculosis
conjunctiva	induration	tine test

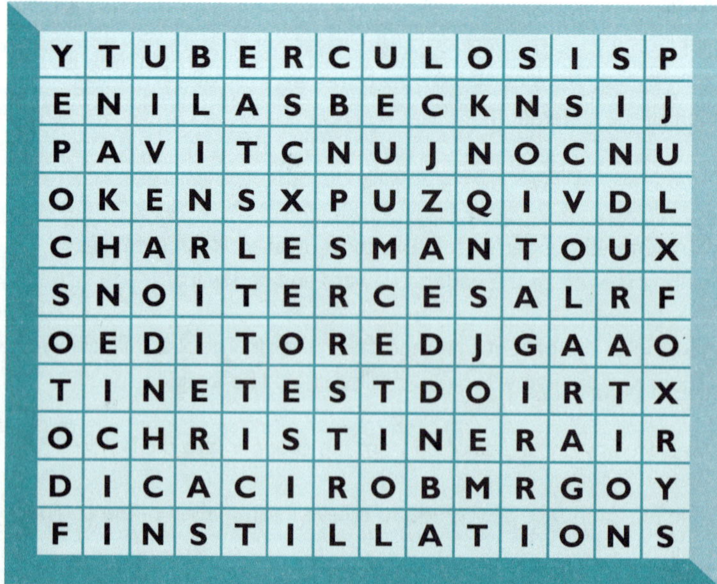

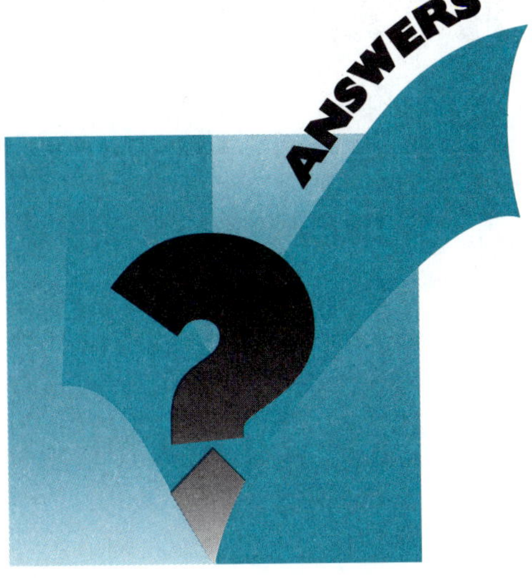

Vocabulary

1. i	5. m	9. g	13. o
2. n	6. b	10. l	14. h
3. f	7. k	11. e	15. d
4. c	8. a	12. j	16. p

Student Activities

1. Answers may vary.

2. Answers may vary.

3. Complete Conversion Table

LIQUID MEASURE		**WEIGHT**	
Metric	Approximate Apothecary Equivalents	Metric	Approximate Apothecary Equivalents
250 mL	8 fluid ounces	30 grams	1 fluid ounce
30 mL	1 fluid ounce	3 g	45 grams
2 g	30 grains ($^1/_2$ dram)	6 mg	$^1/_{10}$ grain
1000 mL	1 quart	1.5 mg	$^1/_{40}$ grain
100 mL	$3^1/_2$ fluid ounces	1.5 g	22 grains

4. Answers may vary.

Discussion Topics

1. PPD is the referred test for tuberculin testing because of its degree of accuracy and reliability. A healthcare worker found to have a positive test result must receive treatment. TB is a reportable communicable disease. TB is easily transmitted to patients and family

2. Answers may vary.

Review and Rationale

1. This stabilizes the patient's arm in case he/she jerks from the sting of the tine unit.

2. Sufficient pressure must be exerted on the disc so that four puncture sites and a circular depression from the plastic base are made visible on the patient's skin when the tine unit is removed.

3. The physician must be notified if the patient had drainage or any complications from previous irrigations so he/she can determine whether treatment should be continued.

4. This position allows the irrigation solution to flow from the ear into the basin.

5. Care must be taken not to obstruct the opening of the ear canal with the syringe tip.

6. Discontinue irrigation and notify the physician.

7. Eye movement helps to distribute the medication over the eyeball.

8. If the tube does touch the eyelid, it is considered contaminated and must be discarded unless it is being used by only one patient.

9. As a medical assistant, you must always be sure that you are administering the right drug, at the right dose, by the right route, at the right time, to the right patient.

10. Eyes and ears are delicate organs which must be treated gently.

Multiple Choice

1. c	3. d	5. a	7. c	9. e
2. d	4. d	6. c	8. a	10. c

True or False

1. T	3. F	5. F	7. F	9. F
2. T	4. T	6. F	8. T	10. T

Word Puzzle

HISTORICAL HIGHLIGHTS

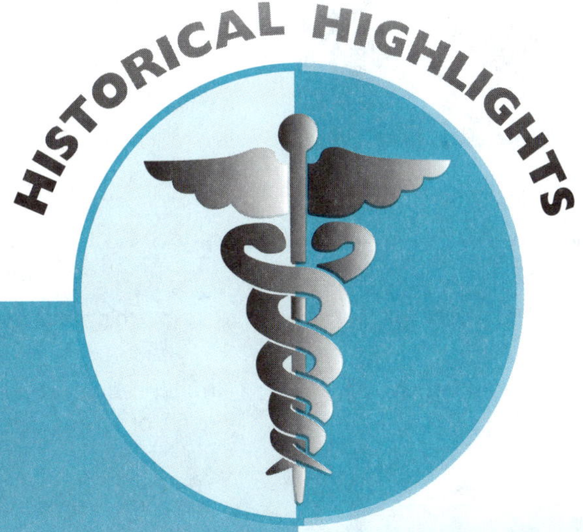

It was William Harvey (1578-1657), an English *anatomist,* who believed blood circulated through the body in only one direction. He predicted it passed from vessels known as arteries to *veins* through *capillaries.* This was proven in 1661 by Marcello Malpighi (1628–1694) by use of the *microscope.* This instrument enabled scientists to examine and study *bacteria* and *microorganisms.* However, the true significance of these microscopic lifeforms was not recognized until 150 years later.

As a medical assistant, you will often collect specimens from patients, process them in the office laboratory, or send them to an outside facility for testing. Your use and understanding of the microscope is essential in processing the specimens. The results of these tests will help the physician to determine an accurate diagnosis and treatment for the patient. As your skills increase in these areas, your professional effectiveness will be enhanced.

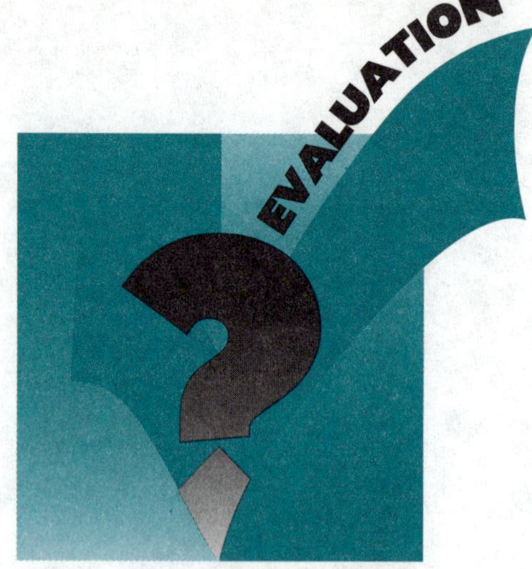

Vocabulary

Write the letter of each term on the line of its matching definition at the right.

a. source-oriented format

b. integrated system

c. problem oriented system

d. subjective findings

e. objective findings

f. assessment

g. plan

h. centrifuge

i. microscope

j. urinalysis

k. specific urine gravity

l. reagent strip

m. supernatant fluid

n. 10x eyepiece

o. chemical examination of urine

1. _____ motorized device separates liquids into components of varying densities by spinning them at high speeds

2. _____ compares weight of urine with an equal amount of distilled water to measure how concentrated the specimen is

3. _____ observations or measurement by the examiners

4. _____ complete examination of urine

5. _____ plastic strip impregnated with various chemicals

6. _____ contains all information such as office visits and treatments given, in strict chronological order

7. _____ fluid remaining at the top of the tube after urine is centrifuged

8. _____ file all report slips on pre-printed forms chronologically according to the specialty

9. _____ statement made by the patient

10. _____ checking for pH, protein, glucose, Ketone, bilirubin, nitrate, urobilinogen, and blood in the urine

11. _____ lowest power objective

12. _____ evaluation of the patient's status

13. _____ system consisting of the data base, problem list, plan, and progress note

14. _____ instrument used in the laboratory to magnify tiny objects

15. _____ method prescribed for treatment of patient such as diagnostic, therapeutic, or educational means

Student Activities

1. Using Figure 9-1 for reference, compare the microscope in your classroom with this illustration. Note the similar pieces as well as any variations between the two.

2. Consider the reporting of sensitive test results (ie. blood alcohol, HIV, controlled substances, and surgical pathology). Research the required and accepted procedure for reporting these test results. Who may receive the results? What identification must be furnished? When may these be given to someone other than the patient?

3. Alcohol, urine, and drug abuse testing by law enforcement agencies require consent signed by the person being tested before any specimens are collected. The patient has the right to refuse to sign a consent. If the testing is refused or the patient does not comply

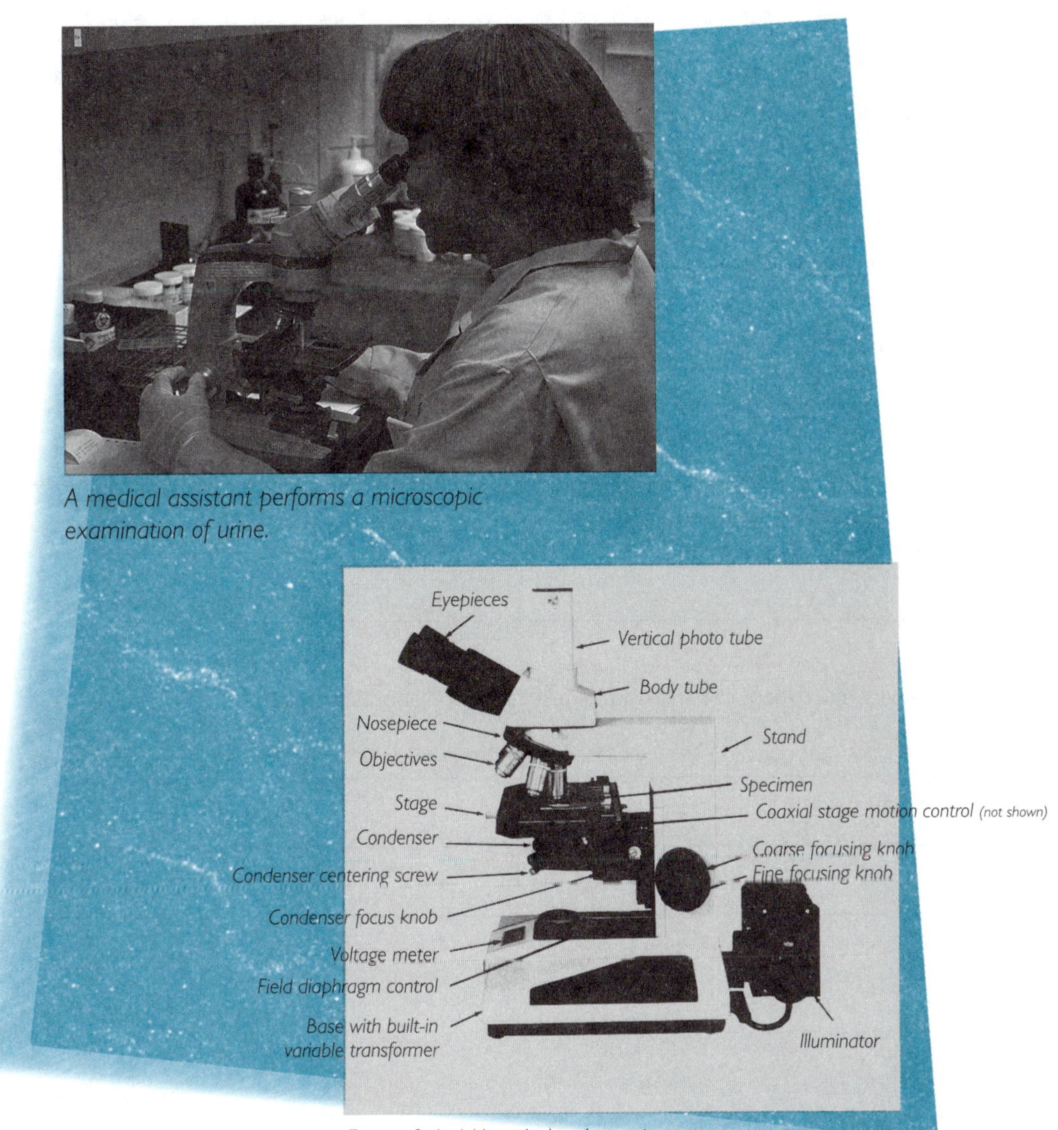

A medical assistant performs a microscopic examination of urine.

Figure 9-1 Nikon Labophot microscope.

with the controlled urine collection, that will be documented on a Chain of Custody (CC) form. This is also called a chain of possession. It traces the transfer of the specimen from one person to another if used to provide a legally defensible record of the specimen handling. Check with your local hospital laboratory or outside laboratory facility for guidelines in collecting such specimens. Also, research confidentiality of test results.

Discussion Topics

1. A test may be considered "stat" if the results will be used to directly and immediately affect the management or therapy provided for the patient. Discuss how and when a "stat" order is handled.

2. A patient reports to a laboratory and requests a test be performed without a written request from a licensed practitioner. Under what circumstances can the test be performed?

3. If the patient calls for a laboratory report, how should the medical assistant handle the request?

Review and Rationale

Answer the following questions in the space provided.

1. Why use a separate lab requisition for each test requested for your collected specimen?

____

____

____

2. Why must you know the normal test ranges of laboratory results?

____

____

____

3. Why is a circle or red underline used on laboratory test results?

____

____

____

4. Why do physicians usually sign or put a check on a laboratory report?

____

____

____

5. Why file all lab reports together with the latest information on top?

____

____

____

6. Why use xylene and lens tissue to clean the microscope lens?

____

____

____

7. Why adjust the light by raising or lowering the substage condenser and by opening or closing the diaphragm?

____

____

____

8. Why not force a high-powered objective on a microscope slide?

____

____

____

9. Why is the specific gravity of urine important?

____

____

____

10. Why do reagent strips change color when dipped in urine?

____

____

____

11. Why should you check your watch at the exact time you remove the reagent strip from the urine?

____

____

____

12. Why should you avoid touching the bottom of the test tube after adding the Clinitest tablet?

____

____

____

13. Why is the reagent strip method the most practical for use in a physician's office or clinic?

____

____

____

Performance Test

In a skills laboratory, a simulation of a job-like environment the medical assistant student must demonstrate skill and knowledge in performing the following procedures without reference to source materials. Time limits for the performance of each procedure are to be assigned by the instructor.

1. chemical urinalysis
2. Clinitest
3. bacteriology examination

You are expected to perform the above activities with 100% accuracy 90% of the time (9 out of 10 times).

Performance Checklist

DIRECTIONS: The following checklist will be used to evaluate your performance of each procedure.

Checklist 9-1: Chemical examination using reagent strips (See Figure 9-2 A–C)

Checklist	S or NA	U	NO	Comment
1. Dip the test areas of the strip into a freshly voided urine specimen.				
2. Remove the strip immediately and gently tap it on the side of the specimen container.				
3. Check your watch at the exact time you remove the strip from the specimen container.				
4. Compare the test areas on the strip to the appropriate color chart on the bottle at the times specified.				
5. Record the results of each test reading.				

*S or NA = satisfactory or not applicable; U = unsatisfactory; NO = not observed

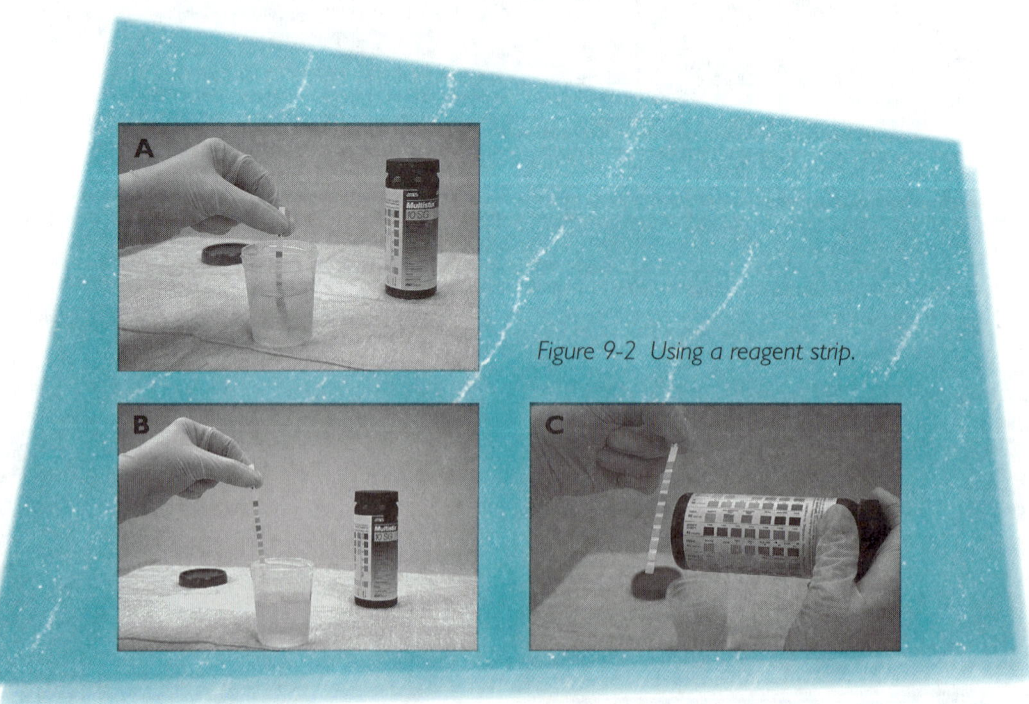

Figure 9-2 Using a reagent strip.

Checklist 9-2: Performance of the Clinitest (Figure 9-3)

Checklist	S or NA	U	NO	Comment
1. Place 5 drops of urine into the test tube and rinse the dropper.				
2. Add 10 drops of water and one Clinitest tablet.				
3. After the boiling reaction is complete, wait 15 seconds and shake the tube gently.				
4. Compare the color of the contents with the tablet bottle color chart.				
5. After completing the test, record the results.				

*S or NA = satisfactory or not applicable; U = unsatisfactory; NO = not observed

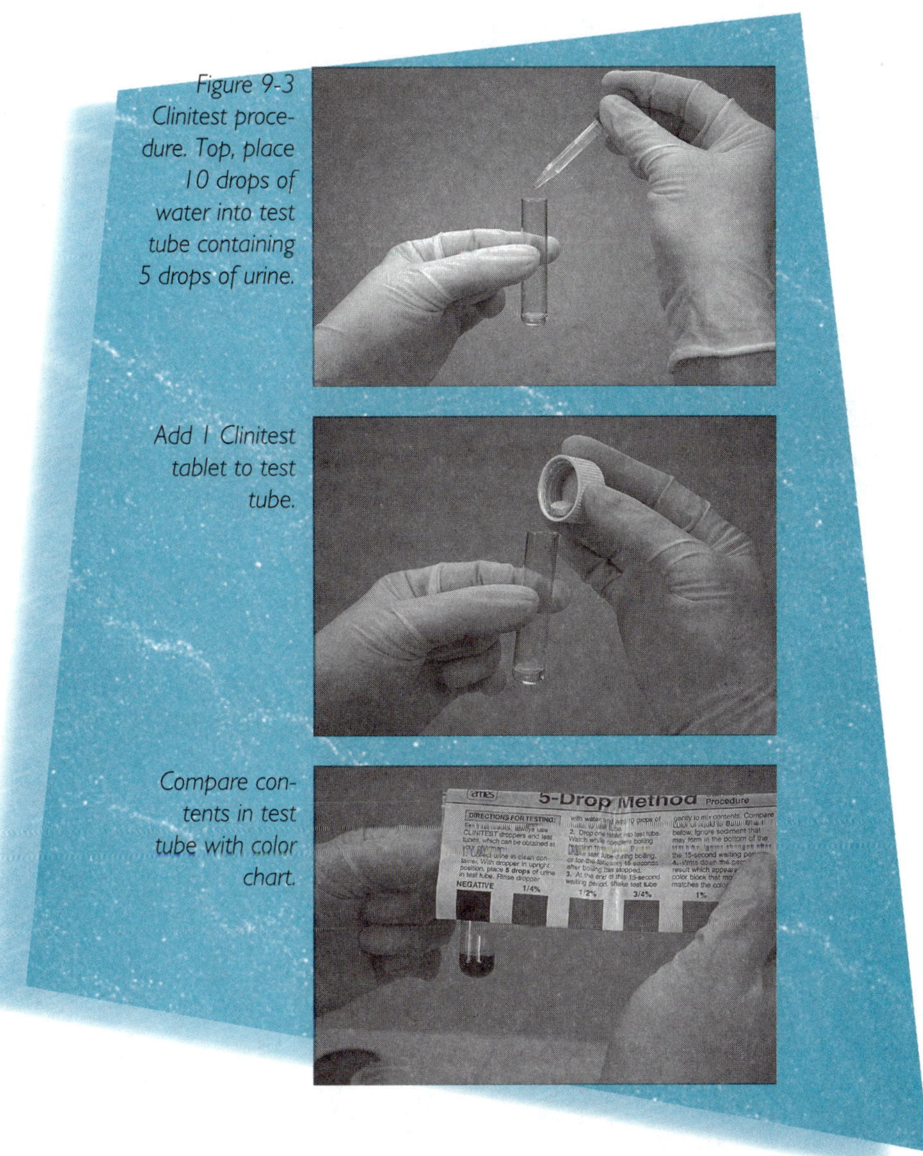

Figure 9-3 Clinitest procedure. Top, place 10 drops of water into test tube containing 5 drops of urine.

Add 1 Clinitest tablet to test tube.

Compare contents in test tube with color chart.

Checklist 9-3: Bacteriology Examination

Checklist	S or NA	U	NO	Comment
1. Remove the strip from the wrapper.				
2. Dip it in the urine specimen for five seconds and remove.				
3. Note time on your watch and read the nitrite test area 30 seconds later.				
4. Insert the strip in the sterile plastic pouch and seal.				
5. Incubate the pouch 12-18 hours				
6. Read results without removing the strip from the transparent pouch.				
7. Compare the color densities on both the culture pads with the chart provided.				
8. Record the results and dispose of the still-sealed pouch by incineration.				
9. Upon completion of the urinalysis procedure, discard the specimen and the Reagent strips in the appropriate places for contaminated materials.				
10. Sterilize all test tubes and disinfect laboratory machines according to office and manufacturer policies.				
11. Disinfect work area.				

*S or NA = satisfactory or not applicable; U = unsatisfactory; NO = not observed

Multiple Choice

From the options listed under each question or statement, select the correct answer or answers. Write the corresponding letter or letters in the answer space.

1. Changes in the chemical or physical characteristics of body fluids, such as _______________, offers clues about the patient's health:
   a. blood and urobilinogen
   b. blood or urine
   c. hematocrit and hemoglobin
   d. bilirubin and urine

2. The specimen container must be labeled with the following: _______
   a. date
   b. time specimen was collected
   c. patient's name
   d. physician's name
   e. all of the above

3. Name the three basic formats for organizing a patient's file: _______
   a. subjective, objective, assessment
   b. source-oriented, integrated, and problem oriented
   c. integrated problem list, source-oriented, POMR
   d. subjective, objective, plan

4. To maintain a source-oriented format, file all report slips on pre-printed forms: _______
   a. chronologically according to the specialty
   b. in strict chronological order
   c. by subject
   d. in the order they are received

5. To clean the objective lens of the microscope, use: _______
   a. alcohol wipes
   b. xylene and lens tissue
   c. glass polish
   d. none of the above

6. To adjust the light on the microscope: _______
   a. attach the 10x eyepiece
   b. use high-powered objective
   c. use coarse-focusing knob
   d. lower or raise substage condenser

7. To make the field of vision clear while using the microscope, use the: _______
   a. substage condenser
   b. fine focus adjustment
   c. a microscope slide
   d. close the diaphragm

8. The urinalysis is divided into four categories: _______
   a. general physical characteristics, chemical and microscopic examinations, and the detection of bacteria
   b. color, bilirubin, centrifuging, detection of bacteria
   c. appearance, chemical examination, bacteria and casts
   d. physical characteristics, centrifuged urine sediment examination, and protein

9. Physical characteristics of the freshly voided urine specimen may indicate presence of disorders such as: _______
   a. renal disease
   b. bladder or urinary tract infection
   c. tumors
   d. hepatitis and congested heart failure
   e. all of the above

10. How should urine smell? _______
    a. fruity
    b. putrid
    c. odorless
    d. acidic

11. The normal appearance of a urine specimen should be: _______
    a. cloudy
    b. opaque
    c. clear
    d. translucent
    e. none of the above

12. What is the average adult urinary output? _______
    a. 725–1500 milliliters per day
    b. 750–2000 milliliters per day
    c. 775–2250 milliliters per day
    d. 700–2500 milliliters per day

13. Excessive urination may indicate: _______
    a. diabetes mellitus
    b. diabetes insipidus
    c. dehydration
    d. none of the above

14. Polyuria, too little urination, may be a sign of: _______
    a. congestive heart disease
    b. diabetes insipidus
    c. liver failure
    d. severe dehydration

15. Normal specific gravity is between: _______
    a. 1.005 and 1.030
    b. 1 and 1.005
    c. 1.025 and 1.030
    d. none of the above

16. Abnormally low specific gravity may indicate: _______
    a. present of diabetes insipidus
    b. pyelonephritis
    c. various kidney anomalies
    d. none of the above

17. Abnormally high specific gravity values may be a sign of: _______
    a. diabetes mellitus
    b. congested heart failure
    c. hepatic diseases
    d. adrenal insufficiency
    e. all of the above
    f. none of the above

18. The presence of a large number of red and white blood cells plus a few epithelial cells may indicate: _______
    a. hemorrhagic diseases
    b. infection
    c. generation of the renal tubules
    d. all of the above

19. The progress note section of the record keeping system is divided into which four parts: _______
    a. lab, x ray, H&P, and health survey
    b. problem list, lab, history, and physical
    c. subjective, objective, assessment, and plan
    d. integrated medical record system

20. Use the Microstix-3 test for the presence of: _______
    a. nitrates
    b. bacteria
    c. gram-negative bacteria
    d. none of the above

True or False

Determine whether each of the following statements is true or false. Check the box marked T or F at the left of the statement.

T F

☐ ☐ 1. Laboratories immediately report test results to you by telephone.

☐ ☐ 2. You only need to notify the physician of verbal reports of laboratory specimens.

☐ ☐ 3. File all laboratory reports as soon as they arrive.

☐ ☐ 4. A patient's file should be organized to provide easy viewing and assessment of information.

☐ ☐ 5. Most laboratories mail test results.

☐ ☐ 6. Record telephoned information accurately and label the slip as a verbal report and notify the physician of the findings.

☐ ☐ 7. Never file a report before the physician has reviewed it.

☐ ☐ 8. A source-oriented format consists of all information in strict chronological order.

☐ ☐ 9. The P in SOAP (plan) states what is done to solve the problems.

☐ ☐ 10. Through centrifugal force, heavy or solid components of liquid move to the bottom of the specimen tube.

☐ ☐ 11. The centrifuge is calibrated and cleaned annually.

☐ ☐ 12. The presence of glucose in the urine may be determined by using the Reagent strip.

☐ ☐ 13. There are five color blocks on the Clinitest bottle ranging from violet to amber.

☐ ☐ 14. An orange reading of the Clinitest indicates a large amount of glucose present in the urine.

☐ ☐ 15. The fluid remaining at the top of the tube of centrifuged urine is known as supernatant fluid.

Word Puzzle

Complete the puzzle using the following medical terminology definitions related to laboratory orientation and urinalysis.

ACROSS

1. states what is done to solve the problem
3. instrument used to magnify tiny objects
4. statements made by the patient
5. evaluation of the patient's status
6. observed of measured findings by the examiner
7. motorized device which spins at high speeds
8. the act of unifying or bringing together

DOWN

1. consists of: data base, problem list, the plan, and progress notes
2. filed chronologically according to specialty

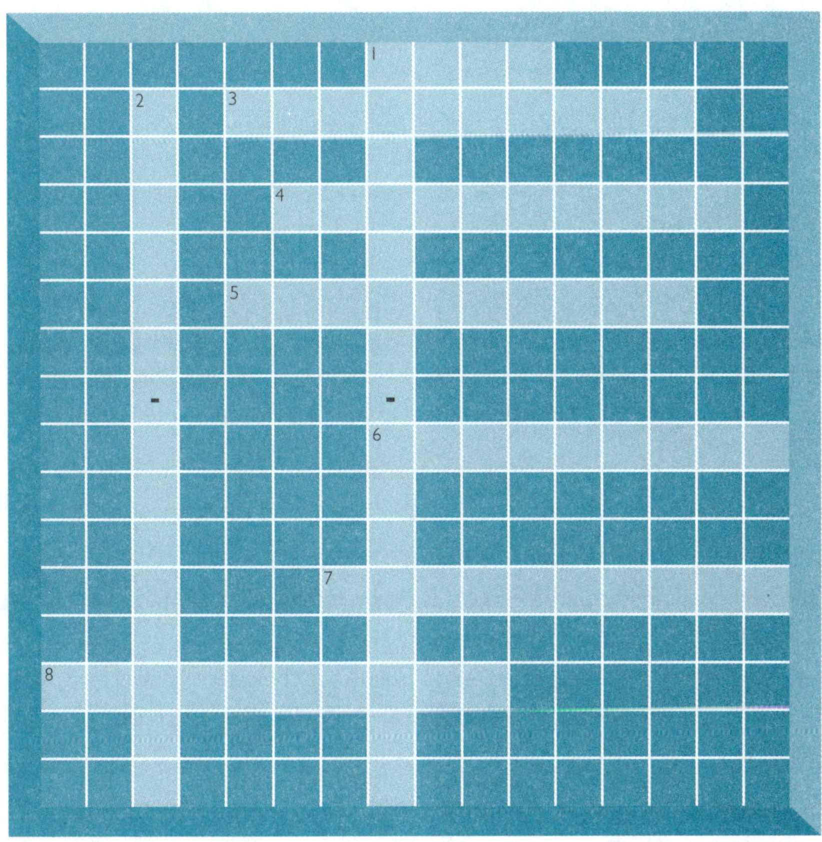

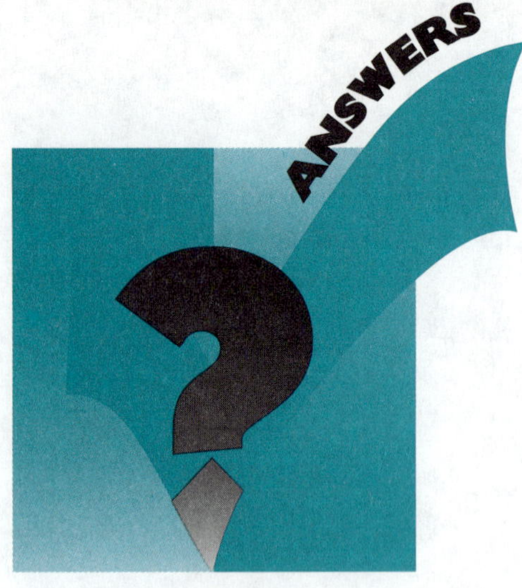

Vocabulary

1. h	4. j	7. m	10. o	13. c
2. k	5. l	8. a	11. n	14. i
3. e	6. b	9. d	12. f	15. g

Student Activities

1–3. Answers may vary.

Discussion Topics

1. "Stat" procedures are handled within the laboratory on a "time of arrival" basis. At certain times of the day there may be a large number of specimens awaiting "stat" analysis. Use discretion in order to hold to a minimum the number of procedures requested "stat".

2. Answers may vary. One example may be that the laboratory will perform tests without a written request from a licensed practitioner or other authorized agent under the following specific conditions:

   a. a properly documented verbal request is received from a licensed practitioner

   b. a screening test is performed. The results are not reported to a licensed practitioner. Presently such testing is limited to glucose or cholesterol testing programs and over-the-counter tests (i.e. pregnancy, glucose, and chemical urinalysis).

3. Answers may vary. One possibility is if the physician has authorized the medical assistant to report to the patient, the report will be given directly to the patient (if non-sensitive). Before giving a report by telephone, the patient will be asked for his/her social security number and other data as an identity check. If the physician is not available and/or the patient insists, a report may be given verbally. Only the results will be given. Normal range or interpretation should not be given.

Review and Rationale

1. Because tests are usually examined in different areas of the lab, most laboratories provide specific requisition forms for each test performed.

2. You must know the normal test ranges so that you can immediately report abnormalities to the physician.

3. A circle or red underline brings abnormal test results to the physician's attention quickly.

4. Physicians usually sign or put a check on a laboratory report after it is reviewed. You may then file the report in the patient's medical record.

5. You must know the normal test ranges so that you can immediately report abnormalities to the physician.

6. Placing the latest information on top is most important for the patient's current care and treatment.

7. Using xylene and lens tissue protects the lens from damage and makes it clean.

8. Adjusting the light by raising or lowering the substage condenser and by opening or closing the diaphragm gives you a clear, distinct field.

9. Forcing a high-powered objective on a microscope slide may break the slide, scratch the objective, or damage the lens.

10. The degree of urine concentration helps to determine the kidney's ability to filter out waste products.

11. The reagent strip is a plastic strip with up to ten pieces of colored, filtered paper attached and impregnated with various chemicals. The elements present in the urine sample causes the chemicals to produce a color range indicative of the presence of disease or a normal reading.

12. It is critical that you read each urine test at the proper time.

13. Avoid touching the bottom of the test tube when the Clinitest tablet is added to the specimen as heat is generated during the boiling reaction.

14. The reagent strip method is the most practical for use in a physician's office or clinic because it does not require special facilities, and personnel seem to prefer the culture method.

Multiple Choice

1. b	5. b	9. e	13. a	17. e
2. e	6. d	10. d	14. d	18. d
3. c	7. b	11. c	15. a	19. c
4. a	8. a	12. b	16. d	20. d

True or False

1. F	4. T	7. T	10. T	13. F
2. F	5. F	8. F	11. F	14. T
3. F	6. T	9. T	12. F	15. T

Word Puzzle

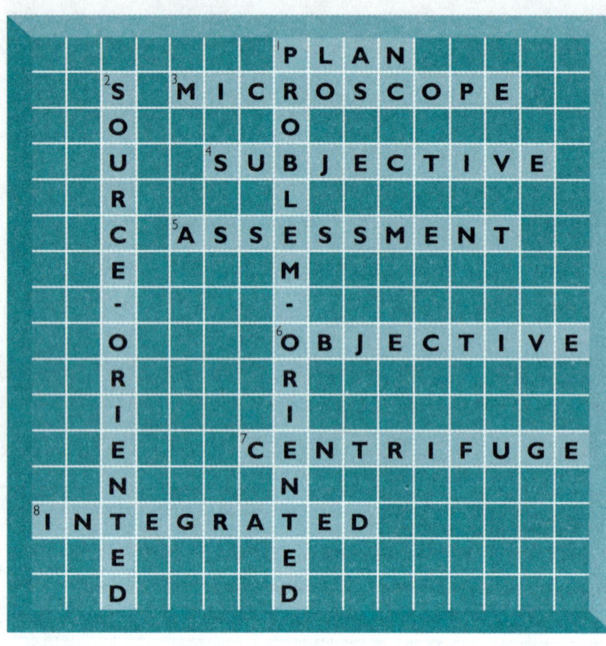

HISTORICAL HIGHLIGHTS

Hematology is the study and science concerned with blood and blood-forming tissues. The word begins with the Greek prefix *hemato-* indicating blood. Hemorrhage was of primary concern following injury. Methods to control bleeding include: tourniquets, sutures, and crushed roots and leaves. Using ice and snow to control bleeding, Hippocrates (460-377) observed the analgesic action of temperature as a therapeutic entity. Hot irons were also used to coagulate blood. The stoppage of blood flow is the result of clotting, taking place by an enzyme reaction that occurs in several stages. This process is known as hemostasis. Prothrombin reacts with thromboplastin and along with other elements form thrombin. The thrombin combines with fibrinogen to form fibrin which is the material of blood clots.

The study of blood and its chemical properties has given rise to various mechanical methods of hemostasis such as the blood-pressure cuff that can be used as a tourniquet, rubber tubing, pressure dressing, and packing. Hemostasis can also be achieved by application of heat or cold to body tissues. The development of cryosurgery to locally freeze diseased tissue permits the frozen tissue to be removed without significant bleeding. Hypothermia, the process of cooling the body to lower temperatures, decreases cellular metabolism and decreases the tissues need for oxygen, thus decreasing bleeding. Electrocautery employs an electric current to coagulate or destroy tissue on contact and sear or seal the tissues, limiting bleeding.

Understanding this information will allow you to more effectively explain procedures to patients and recognize normal and abnormal test values and promote better communication with the laboratory performing your tests.

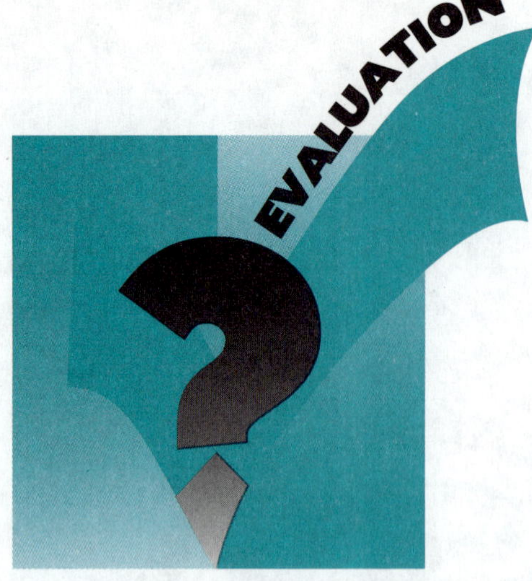

MOSBY'S MEDICAL ASSISTING VIDEO WORKBOOK

Vocabulary

Write the letter of each term on the line of its matching definition at the right.

a. hematology

b. milking

c. diabetes

d. antecubital space

e. blood

f. patent

g. cephalic

h. engorgement

i. dextrostix

j. vacutainer

k. CBC

l. hemoglobin test

m. basilic

n. WBC

o. venipuncture

1. _____ in front of the elbow

2. _____ presence of these helps determine which disease is present

3. _____ rubbing the finger to promote circulation

4. _____ a reagent strip used to check blood glucose

5. _____ vascular congestion

6. _____ large vein, inner side biceps

7. _____ study of blood

8. _____ system to transfer the blood into tubes

9. _____ test performed to determine the oxygen-carrying ability of the blood

10. _____ river of life

11. _____ open wide

12. _____ process to collect larger samples of blood for testing

13. _____ metabolic disease

14. _____ complete blood count

15. _____ pertaining to the head

Student Activities

1. Blood chemistry screens are tests performed on blood to determine values of any numbers of factors. Find the normal values of the following:

    a. calcium

    b. phosphorus

    c. creatinine

    d. uric acid

    e. cholesterol for your age group/gender

    f. total protein

    g. alkaline phosphatase for your age group/gender

    h. glucose

    i. blood urea nitrogen

    j. sodium

2. In the USA, regulations for the collection, storage, and transportation of blood and its components have been established by a federal regulatory agency. Which agency is it? Are there also state or local health authorities which govern the above? What roles do the American National Red Cross and the American Association of Blood Banks play in their respective systems?

3. Clinical Laboratory Improvement Amendments (CLIA) established three categories of laboratory tests: certificate of waiver tests, tests of moderate complexity, and tests of high complexity. Contact the AAMA (American Association of Medical Assistants) executive office for detailed excerpts of the laboratory personnel standards on federal regulations' impact on medical assistants performing laboratory tests.

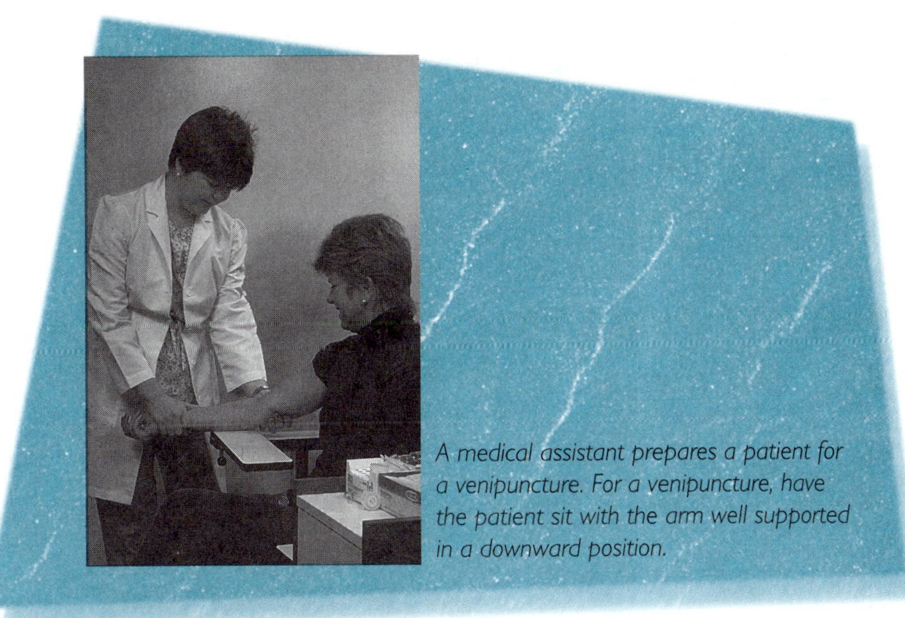

A medical assistant prepares a patient for a venipuncture. For a venipuncture, have the patient sit with the arm well supported in a downward position.

Discussion Topics

1. AIDS is a fatal virus. As a medical assistant, you must protect yourself at all times from exposure. This added caution on your part in turn protects those you come into contact with such as coworkers and, of course, patients. There are many activities that increase risk factors for AIDS—namely, unprotected sexual contact and illicit drug usage—but consider some of the most common false fears about exposure to AIDS. Discuss the following "false fears": mosquitoes, casual contact, and bites by angry individuals.

2. AIDS testing deserves the attention of all health professionals. What is the ELISA test?

3. Double-ended needles for ease in specimen collection are most routinely used for venipuncture. However, the vacuum tubes are nonsterile and backflow of blood from the filled tube to the vein may occur, permitting the entry of bacteria. Discuss maneuvers that may help to avoid such infection.

Review and Rationale

Answer the following questions in the space provided.

1. Why is blood often referred to as the river of life?

____

____

____

2. Why are many studies done on blood?

____

____

____

3. Why should a sturdy arm support be provided for a patient prior to obtaining a blood specimen?

____

____

____

4. Why should you gently rub the finger along the sides prior to a finger stick?

____

____

____

5. Why should the first drop of blood be wiped away following a finger stick?

____

____

____

6. Why shouldn't you squeeze the finger following puncture?

____

____

____

7. Why select an elastic, resilient, sturdy-walled vein for venipuncture?

____

____

____

8. Why use your nondominant hand to draw the skin over the puncture site until it is tense?

____

____

____

9. Why should you ask the patient to elevate his arm slightly following venipuncture?

____

____

____

10. Why use color-coded rubber stoppers on vacuum specimen tubes?

____

____

____

Performance Test

In a skills laboratory, a simulation of a job-like environment, the medical assistant student must demonstrate skill and knowledge in performing the following procedures without reference to source materials. Times limits for the performance of each procedure are to assigned by the instructor.

1. Obtain blood specimens through a fingertip skin puncture and venipuncture.
2. Give normal values for blood glucose levels.

You are expected to perform the above activities with 100% accuracy 90% of the time (9 out of 10 times).

Performance Checklist

DIRECTIONS: The following checklist will be used to evaluate your performance of each procedure.

Checklist 10-1: Obtaining a blood specimen through fingertip skin puncture (See Figure 10-1) and using a reagent strip to determine blood glucose level.

Checklist	S or NA	U	NO	Comment
1. Wash your hands.				
2. Position patient and explain procedure.				
3. Load the automatic blood sampling pen with a sterile lancet. Remove the plastic cap and insert the lancet.				
4. Put on gloves.				
5. Select, clean, and allow puncture site to dry.				
6. Gently rub finger.				
7. Hold the end of the automatic sampling pen and twist off lancet protective disk.				
8. Replace disk with sampling pen's plastic cap.				
9. Grasp patient's finger and position sampling pen's cap over selected skin area.				
10. Press release button and wipe away first drop of blood.				
11. Apply gentle pressure above puncture site.				
12. Lightly touch the blood drop to the strip test pad.				
13. Apply pressure to the puncture site with dry sponge.				
14. Remove lancet from automatic blood sampling pen and dispose in sharps container.				
15. Clean automatic pen, put on clean cap, and store properly.				
16. Label blood sample.				
Glucose test procedure using a dextrostix to determine blood glucose level:				
a. After obtaining blood sample above, wait prescribed time.				
b. Hold strip vertically and wash the blood off.				
c. Compare color on the test strip with color chart and determine glucose reading.				

*S or NA = satisfactory or not applicable; U = unsatisfactory; NO = not observed

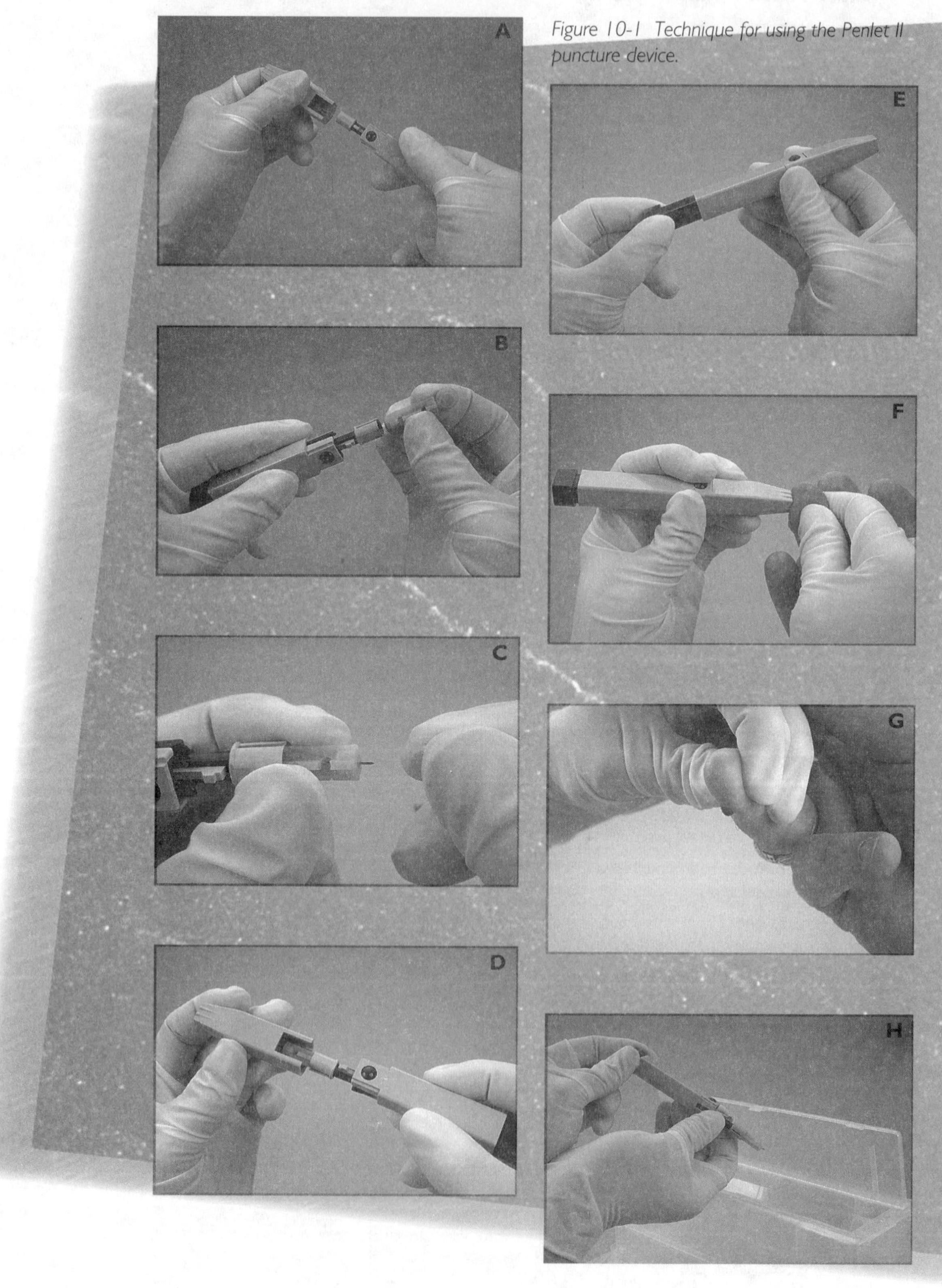

Figure 10-1 Technique for using the Penlet II puncture device.

Checklist 10-2: Venipuncture Procedure using needle and syringe (Figure 10-2)

Checklist	S or NA	U	NO	Comment
1. Select site for venipuncture. Put on disposable single-use exam gloves.				
2. Apply tourniquet and palpate vein.				
3. Swab the venipuncture site.				
4. Remove needle shield and with needle properly positioned perform venipuncture.				
5. Slowly pull back on plunger and release tourniquet.				
6. Place a dry, sterile cotton sponge over puncture site and remove needle.				
7. Apply pressure to site and apply bandaid.				
8. Insert needle into vacutainer.				
9. Dispose of needle and syringe in designated sharps container.				

**S or NA = satisfactory or not applicable; U = unsatisfactory; NO = not observed*

Figure 10-2

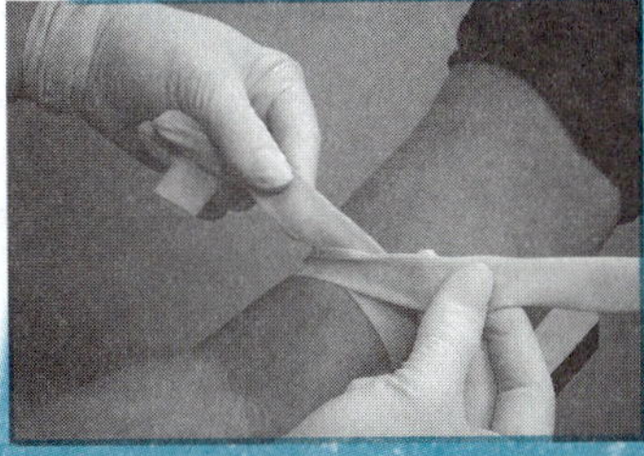
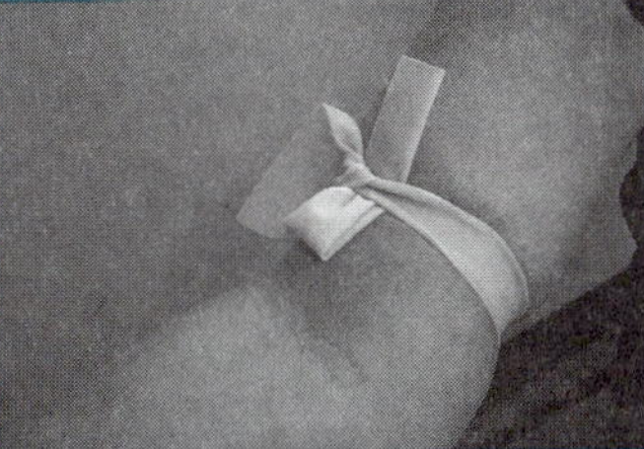
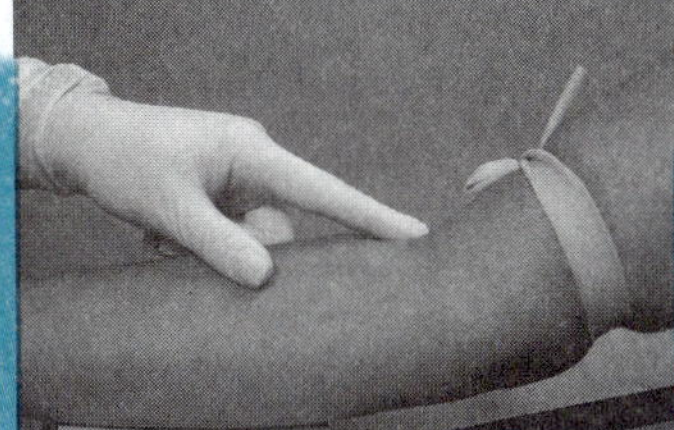

Apply the tourniquet around the patient's arm 3 to 4 inches above the elbow. Cross the ends of the tourniquet and pull the ends away from each other to create tension. Secure the tourniquet by tucking the upper end into the band to form a half-elbow. The tourniquet must be tight enough to obstruct venous blood flow.

Palpate the vein once again after the tourniquet has been positioned.

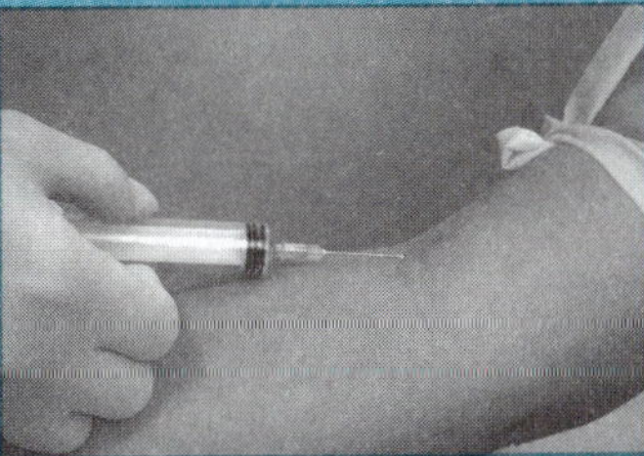
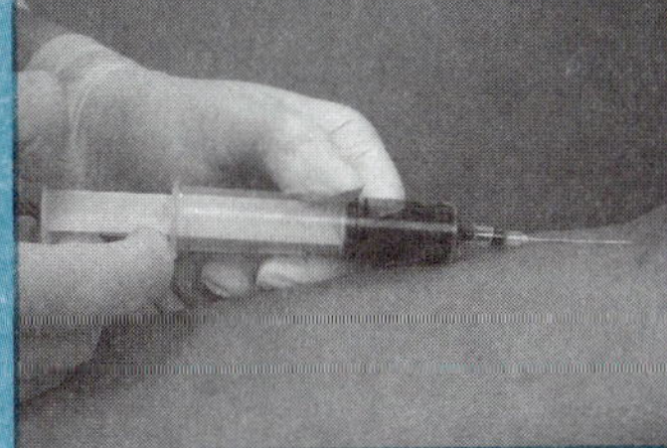
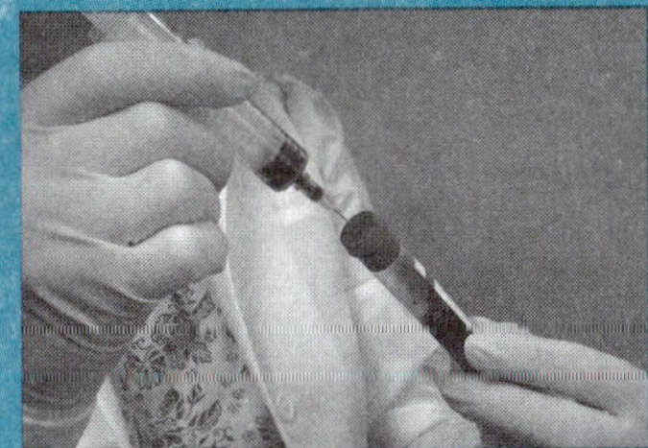

Gently and slowly, insert the needle at a 15-degree angle through the skin into the vein.

After entering the vein, use your nondominant hand to slowly pull on the plunger of the syringe to withdraw blood. Release the tourniquet as soon as blood starts to flow into the syringe.

After obtaining the required amount of blood and removing the needle from the vein, inject blood into the test tube. When using a vacuum tube, leave the needle on the syringe and gently insert the needle through the rubber stopper on the tube.

Multiple Choice

From the options listed under each question or statement, select the correct answer or answers. Write the corresponding letter or letters in the answer space.

1. To obtain a blood specimen by the fingertip skin puncture method, you need: _______
   a. an automatic blood sampling pen
   b. sterile lancet
   c. disposable alcohol sponges
   d. cotton or gauze sponges
   e. disposable gloves
   f. all of the above
   g. all except e

2. If the patient's fingers are cold, do any of the following except: _______
   a. milking
   b. rub them or apply a warm pack
   c. squeeze fingers firmly
   d. ask patient to dangle her hand toward the floor

3. Label blood samples with which of the following: _______
   a. patient's name
   b. physician's name
   c. source of the sample
   d. date and time
   e. all of the above
   f. a,b, and d

4. The most common sites for a venipuncture are all except: _______
   a. basilic
   b. innominate
   c. cephalic
   d. none of the above

5. A vacutainer system contains what gauze needle? _______
   a. 1 1/2" to 2"
   b. 1"
   c. 1" to 1 1/2"
   d. 1 1/2"

6. Labels on the vacuum tubes indicate all of the follow except: _______
   a. contained additive
   b. expiration date
   c. approximate amount of blood drawn into the tube
   d. EDTA

7. Low hemoglobin and hematocrit concentrations may indicate: _________
   a. anemia
   b. recent hemorrhage
   c. fluid retention
   d. all of the above
   e. none of the above

8. High hemoglobin and hematocrit concentrations may suggest all of the following except: _________
   a. fluid retention
   b. dehydration
   c. polycythemia
   d. anemia

9. The normal range of a hematocrit for women is: _________
   a. 12
   b. 33 to 46 percent
   c. 40 to 54 percent
   d. none of the above

10. The normal hemoglobin range for males is between: _________
    a. 14 to 18 gm/100 ml blood
    b. 12 to 16 gm/100 ml blood
    c. 12 to 14 gm/100 ml blood
    d. 14 to 16 gm/100 ml blood

True or False

Determine whether each of the following statements is true or false. Check the box marked T or F at the left of the statement.

T   F

☐ ☐ 1. When performing venipuncture, release the tourniquet as soon as blood begins to fill the tube.

☐ ☐ 2. Remove the tourniquet after removing the needle.

☐ ☐ 3. Remove the tube from the holder before the vacuum is exhausted.

☐ ☐ 4. When drawing blood for blood culture, first draw the tube which contains no additives.

☐ ☐ 5. Blue capped tubes are used for tests performed on whole blood such as coagulation studies.

T   F

☐   ☐   6. Blood specimens must be tested within two hours of collection.

☐   ☐   7. A blood glucose test is one blood test that can be easily performed in the physician's office using a reagent strip.

☐   ☐   8. A normal blood sugar reading is between 80 and 120 mg/100 ml.

☐   ☐   9. Gray capped tubes are used for performing tests on blood glucose and alcohol levels.

☐   ☐   10. Hematocrit and hemoglobin are studied together to help diagnose a patient's condition.

Word Puzzle

Circle the following medical terms related to hematology.

hematology	milking	hemoglobin
venipuncture	glucose	
diabetes	vacutainer	

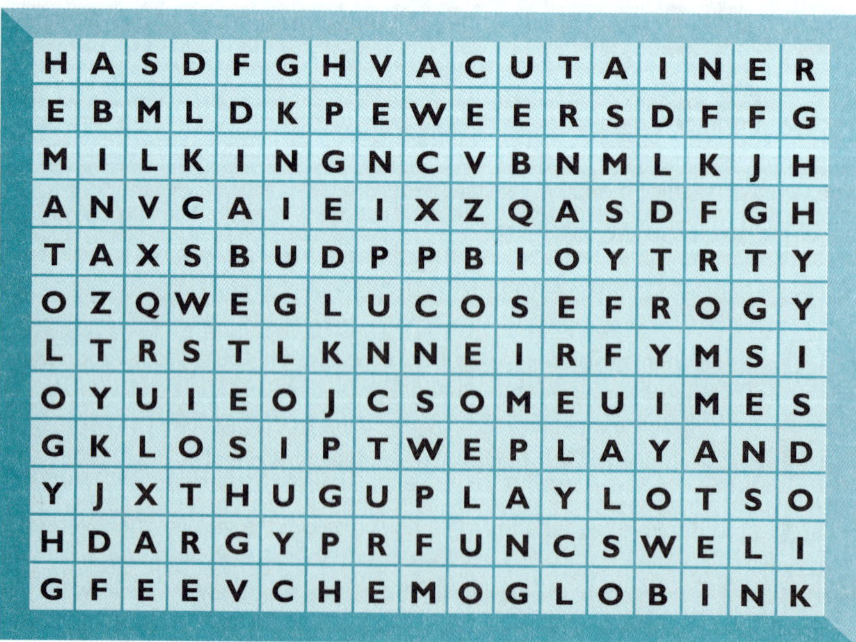

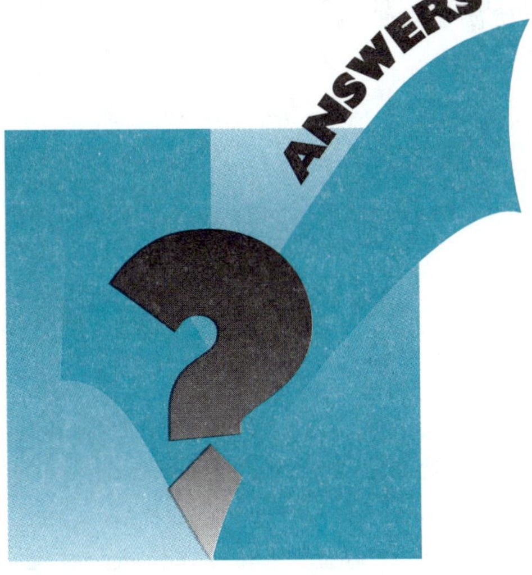

Vocabulary

1. d	4. i	7. a	10. e	13. c
2. n	5. h	8. j	11. f	14. k
3. b	6. m	9. l	12. o	15. g

Student Activities

1. Answers may vary depending on source of reference.

Calcium	8.5 - 10.5 mg/dL
Phosphorus	2.0 - 4.5 mg/dL
Creatinine	0.9 - 1.5 mg/dL
Uric Acid	2.4 - 8.5 mg/dL
Cholesterol	Answers will vary
Total protein	5.90 - 7.70 g/dL
Alkaline phosphatase	Answer will vary
Glucose	72-114 mg/dL
Blood urea nitrogen	4-27 mg/dL
Sodium	137-148 mmol/L

2. Answers may vary, but in general the FDA regulates the collection, storage, and transportation of blood and its components. Local and state agencies may also have regulatory authority. Likewise the American National Red Cross and the American Association of Blood Banks have standards which affect their respective systems. Check your local agencies for reference.

3. It is the medical assistant's responsibility to keep up to date on any regulations governing the practice of medicine delegated to this allied health professional. The excerpts mentioned detail the training, proficiency, and certification required for medical assistants to perform laboratory tests in the physician's office.

Discussion Topics

1. a. There is no credible scientific evidence that mosquitoes spread AIDS. The Centers for Disease Control and Prevention (CDC) and other reputable experts have disputed the claim that mosquitoes transmit AIDS.

   b. Casual contact is not a risk. You do not get AIDS from touching, social kissing, coughing or sneezing. You do not get AIDS from contact with eating utensils, water fountains, toilet seats, telephones, typewriters, and other equipment. You do not get AIDS from using facilities such as public swimming pools, restrooms, or gymnasiums. You do not get AIDS from being close to other people such as on a crowded bus, in a classroom, or restaurant.

   c. There is reasonable concern among parents of school age children and law enforcement officials that an occasion might arise where an infected person would bite an uninfected person. Only if the person doing the biting was bleeding from the mouth and seriously broke the skin of the other person could the virus be passed.

2. Blood products from blood donors are screened by the enzyme-linked immunosorbent assay (ELISA) test to detect the presence of HIV antibodies.

3. Reference source for the following answer is *The Merck Manual*.

   a. Remove the tourniquet well before blood flow into the tube has stopped and preferably before the tube stopper is completely punctured.

   b. Moving the patient's arm during sampling should be avoided since even a few centimeters' elevation after the tube draw is complete may lower venous pressure sufficiently to produce backflow.

   c. No pressure should be exerted on the stopper end of the tube. Whenever possible, sterile tubes or needle and tube arrangements that have a check valve in the system should be used.

Review and Rationale

1. Blood is often referred to as the river of life because it is through this special connective tissue that numerous substances are transported to the cells of our body.

2. Many studies are done on blood to help the physician diagnose the condition of a patient.

3. A well supported arm helps to avoid a jerking movement when the finger stick is made.

4. Gently rubbing the finger along the sides, called milking, promotes circulation.

5. Wipe away the first drop of blood following a needle stick as this contains skin tissue and is unusable for testing.

6. Apply gentle pressure above the puncture site to cause the blood to flow freely, but do not squeeze the finger as this dilutes the blood with tissue fluid and causes inaccurate test results.

7. Do not use a weak-walled, fragile, narrow vein (or a sclerosed vein, even if it looks good). Palpate the area to check that the vein is patent. Weak-walled veins are resistant to pressure; fragile veins are usually narrow.

8. This allows the needle to be inserted more easily and less painfully.

9. Ask the patient to elevate his arm slightly to prevent the blood from oozing at the puncture site.

10. Vacuum specimen tubes have color-coded rubber stoppers which indicate the type of test for which they are best suited.

Multiple Choice

1. f	3. e	5. c	7. d	9. b
2. c	4. c	6. d	8. a & d	10. a

True or False

1. T	3. F	5. T	7. T	9. T
2. F	4. F	6. F	8. T	10. T

Word Puzzle

H A S D F G H V A C U T A I N E R
E B M L D K P E W E E R S D F F G
M I L K I N G N C V B N M L K J H
A N V C A I E I X Z Q A S D F G H
T A X S B U D P P B I O Y T R T Y
O Z Q W E G L U C O S E F R O G Y
L T R S T L K N N E I R F Y M S I
O Y U I E O J C S O M E U I M E S
G K L O S I P T W E P L A Y A N D
Y J X T H U G U P L A Y L O T S O
H D A R G Y P R F U N C S W E L I
G F E E V C H E M O G L O B I N K

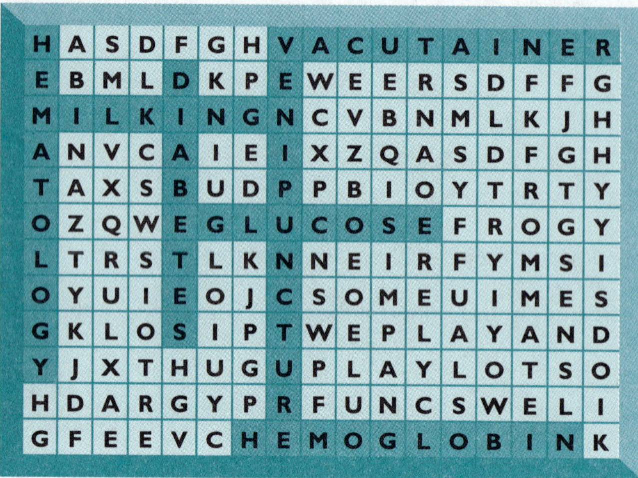

HISTORICAL HIGHLIGHTS

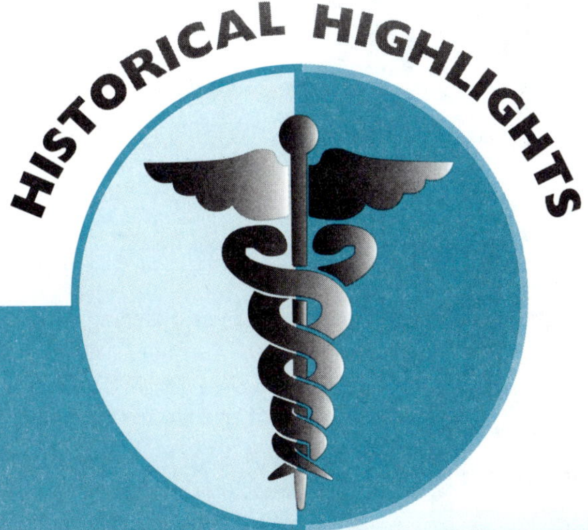

Physical therapy is one division of the specialty of *rehabilitation medicine*. *Occupational therapy* and *speech-language pathology* comprise the other clinical specialties. Medical assistants often perform or assist with *cryotherapy* and *thermotherapy*, two clinical modalities of physical therapy that are used to treat patients with disabilities. Rehabilitation is usually accomplished through *multidisciplinary* endeavor. Physical disabilities is an area of concentration for many physicians, nurses, social workers, therapists, *orthotists, prosthetists,* medical assistants, teachers, engineers, administrators, caretakers, homemakers, and employers.

Everyone working with disabled patients and having the common goal of rehabilitation must have a common knowledge of the principle therapeutic and social concepts of managing disabling conditions.

Many new devices and techniques have been added to physical therapy.

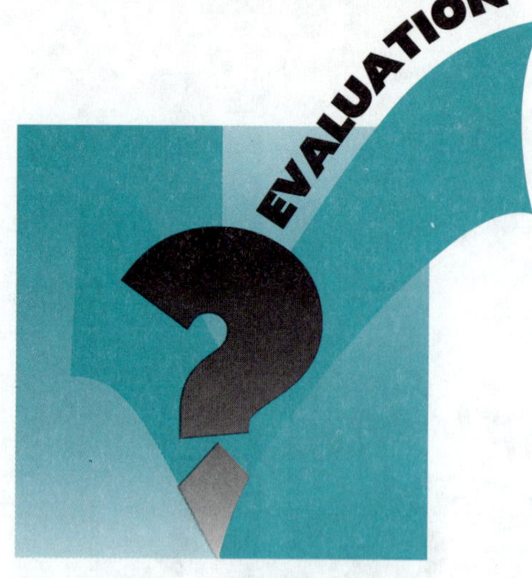

Vocabulary

Write the letter of each term on the line of its matching definition at the right.

a. body mechanics

b. thermotherapy

c. disposable chemical hot pack

d. therapeutic exercise

e. massage

f. extension

g. aquamatic pad

h. rotation

i. flexion

j. abduction

k. cryotherapy

l. adduction

m. chemical cold pack

n. hyperextension

o. ROM

p. supination

q. passive exercises

r. dorsiflexion

s. pronation

t. active resistive exercises

1. _____ exercises designed to assist joint mobility, maintain normal joint, and muscle functioning

2. _____ when a joint is moved so that it closes or the angle between the bones is reduced

3. _____ therapeutic use of cold

4. _____ when a joint is moved so that the joint opens or the angle between the bones increases

5. _____ a systematic and methodical pressure applied to bare skin by the hands

6. _____ when a body part is brought toward the midline

7. _____ the application of heat to the body

8. _____ movement that bends a part backward

9. _____ a pliable device which, when activated, provides heat for a specific amount of time

10. _____ prescribed physical exertion designed to improve one's general health status

11. _____ pliable rubber or plastic flat bag containing a chemical substance and liquid

12. _____ how you use your body when you perform physical actions

13. _____ when a body part is moved away from the midline of the body

14. _____ tubular constructed device filled to about $2/3$ full with distilled water

15. _____ when a limb or part is moved beyond its normal limits

16. _____ movement of the arm to have the palm facing upward

17. _____ exercises performed without any voluntary participation from the patient

18. _____ the process of turning around an axis

19. _____ patient applies pressure or moves a part and the assistant applies resistance to the movement

20. _____ movement of the arm to have the palm facing down

Student Activities

1. The abbreviation ADL stands for Activities of Daily Living. Methods have been developed to appraise, improve, and expand a disabled person's activities so that these activities are comparable to those that are generally carried out by a typical person in his daily routine. In order to be independent within the community, a patient must be able to get in and out of his house unassisted and to use either public or private transportation. Compile a list of obstacles to this independence and then describe an action that could help the patient. Examples to consider include: housekeeping, cooking, and transportation to and from the physician's office.

2. Research the Americans with Disabilities Act and see what impact it might have in the physician's office.

3. Investigate support groups in your community for patients with disabilities.

Discussion Topics

1. Discuss ways in which a disabled patient may have difficulty maneuvering around the physician's office (for example, the rest room, examining room, office, and reception area). What suggestions can be made to accommodate these individuals?

2. The following excerpt is from a case history of a 41-year-old lady who was seen for evaluation because of persistent symptoms following a **MVA:**

> **DISPOSITION:** By history she has a **myofascial strain** of the cervical and lumbar spine. I think she has reached maximum benefits from formal physical therapy and was encouraged to continue with her **AROM** exercises and heat program at the fitness center. For the most part her complaints are not supported by **objective** findings, and I do not think that she should have any significant restrictions in her **ADL** –including doing housework.

Look up any abbreviations or unfamiliar terminology and discuss.

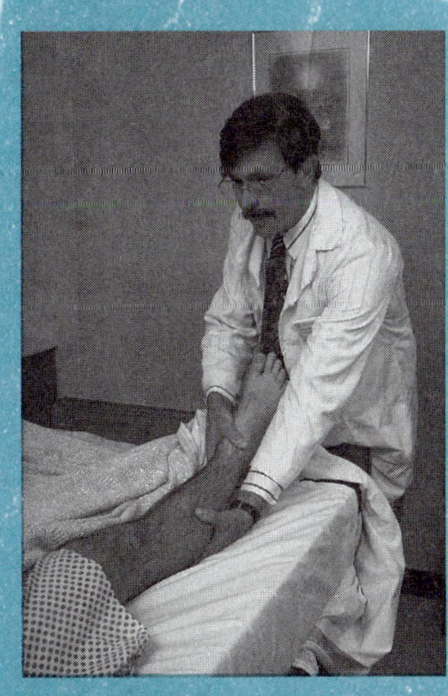

Manual traction is applied by the therapist using the hands to exert a pull on the affected part.

Review and Rationale

Answer the following questions in the space provided.

1. Why should you stand with feet apart and one foot slightly in front of the other?

____

____

____

2. Why should you place one foot on a low stool if you are going to be standing for a long period of time?

____

____

____

3. Why should you keep the heat lamp at least two to four feet away from the skin?

____

____

____

4. Why place an electric heating pad inside a protective covering such as a pillow case before applying it to a dry area?

____

____

____

5. Why should the patient be checked periodically when using cryotherapy?

____

____

____

6. Why cover the thermotherapy pack with a cloth before applying it to the patient's skin?

____

____

____

7. Why should the patient hold the cane on the opposite side of the weakness?

____

____

____

8. Why should a patient be instructed never to lie on an electric heating pad?

____

____

____

9. Why place additional toweling over the ice when using cold or ice packs?

____

____

____

10. Why instruct the patient to always look straight ahead and always rest weight on the palms of the hands, not on the axillary bars of the crutch?

____

____

____

11. Why must the medical assistant assess the patient's exercise capabilities?

____

____

____

12. Why fill a hot water bottle only one-half full and expel the air before putting the top on?

____

____

____

13. Why does the physician assess the patient's disability before prescribing an assistive device?

____

____

____

14. Why is it important to always keep in mind proper body mechanics when transferring a patient to and from the wheelchair?

____

____

____

15. Why remove some of the soaking solution every five minutes or so and add more hot solution?

____

____

____

Performance Test

In a skills laboratory, a simulation of a job-like environment, the medical assistant student must demonstrate skill and knowledge in performing the following procedures without reference to source materials. Time limits for the performance of each procedure are to assigned by the instructor.

1. Transfer a patient from a wheelchair to an examining table.
2. Demonstrate two-, four-, and three-point crutch gait ambulation.
3. Demonstrate instructing a patient in the use of a walker.

You are expected to perform the above activities with 100% accuracy 90% of the time (9 out of 10 times).

Performance Checklist

DIRECTIONS: The following checklist will be used to evaluate your performance of each procedure.

Checklist 11-1: Teaching a Patient About How to Use a Wheelchair (See Figure 11-1)

Checklist	S or NA	U	NO	Comment
Transfer patient from wheelchair to an examining table:				
1. Explain the procedure; lock the brakes, and move the footrests out of the way.				
2. Position a step stool near the examining table.				
3. Ask patient to move forward in the chair; stand facing the patient.				
4. Bend your knees and place your arms under patient's arms using good body mechanics.				
5. Place your hands firmly over the patient's shoulder blades; ask patient to place his hands on your shoulders.				
6. Upon signal, lift upward so patient rises to a standing position.				
7. Ask patient to step onto the stool and pivot so back is to the table.				
8. Ease the patient to a sitting position.				
9. Move patient to a lying position. Raise patient's legs onto the table and lower patient into supine position.				
10. Attend to patient's comfort and safety.				
Transfer patient from examining table into the wheelchair:				
1. Place one arm under the patient's shoulder and your other arm under the knees.				
2. Using a single smooth move, assist the patient to a sitting position.				
3. Using good body mechanics, help patient to move from the table to the wheelchair.				

*S or NA = satisfactory or not applicable; U = unsatisfactory; NO = not observed

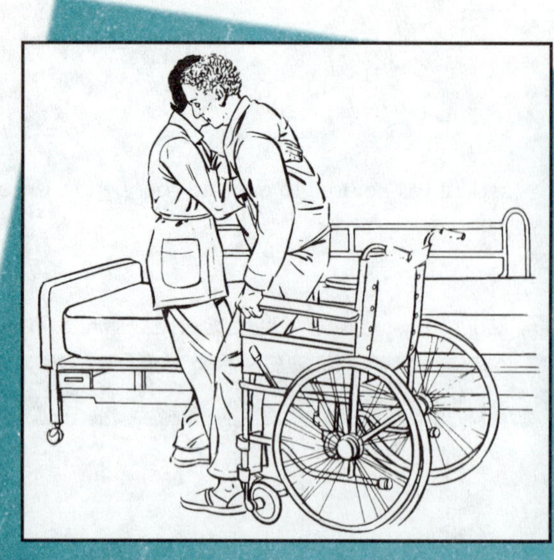

Figure 11-1 The client is helped from the bed to the chair by using a pivoting motion. (From Gerdin: Health Careers Today, St. Louis, 1991, Mosby)

Checklist 11-2: Teaching a Patient How to Use Crutches (See Figure 11-2 A-C)

Checklist	S or NA	U	NO	Comment
Four-point crutch gait ambulation				
1. The right crutch is put forward followed by the left foot.				
2. The left crutch is put forward followed by the right foot.				
3. Repeat action.				
Three-point crutch gait ambulation				
1. Both crutches are advanced forward.				
2. The weaker leg is brought through the crutches followed by the stronger leg.				
3. Sequence repeated.				
Two-point crutch gait ambulation (nonweightbearing)				
1. Both crutches are placed ahead of the patient.				
2. Patient hops forward with one foot.				
Two-point crutch gait ambulation				
1. Alternate feet and crutches move forward together.				
2. Right foot moves forward with the left crutch.				
3. Left foot moves forward with the right crutch.				
4. Sequence repeated.				

*S or NA = satisfactory or not applicable; U = unsatisfactory; NO = not observed

Checklist 11-3: Teaching the Patient to Use a Walker (See Figure 11-3)

Checklist	S or NA	U	NO	Comment
1. Ask patient to stand with the stationary walker positioned slightly in front of him.				
2. Instruct him to shift all weight onto the strong leg as he lifts and advances the walker and the weak leg.				
3. Instruct patient to shift his weight to the walker and the weak leg while moving the strong leg forward.				
4. Repeat sequence.				

*S or NA = satisfactory or not applicable; U = unsatisfactory; NO = not observed

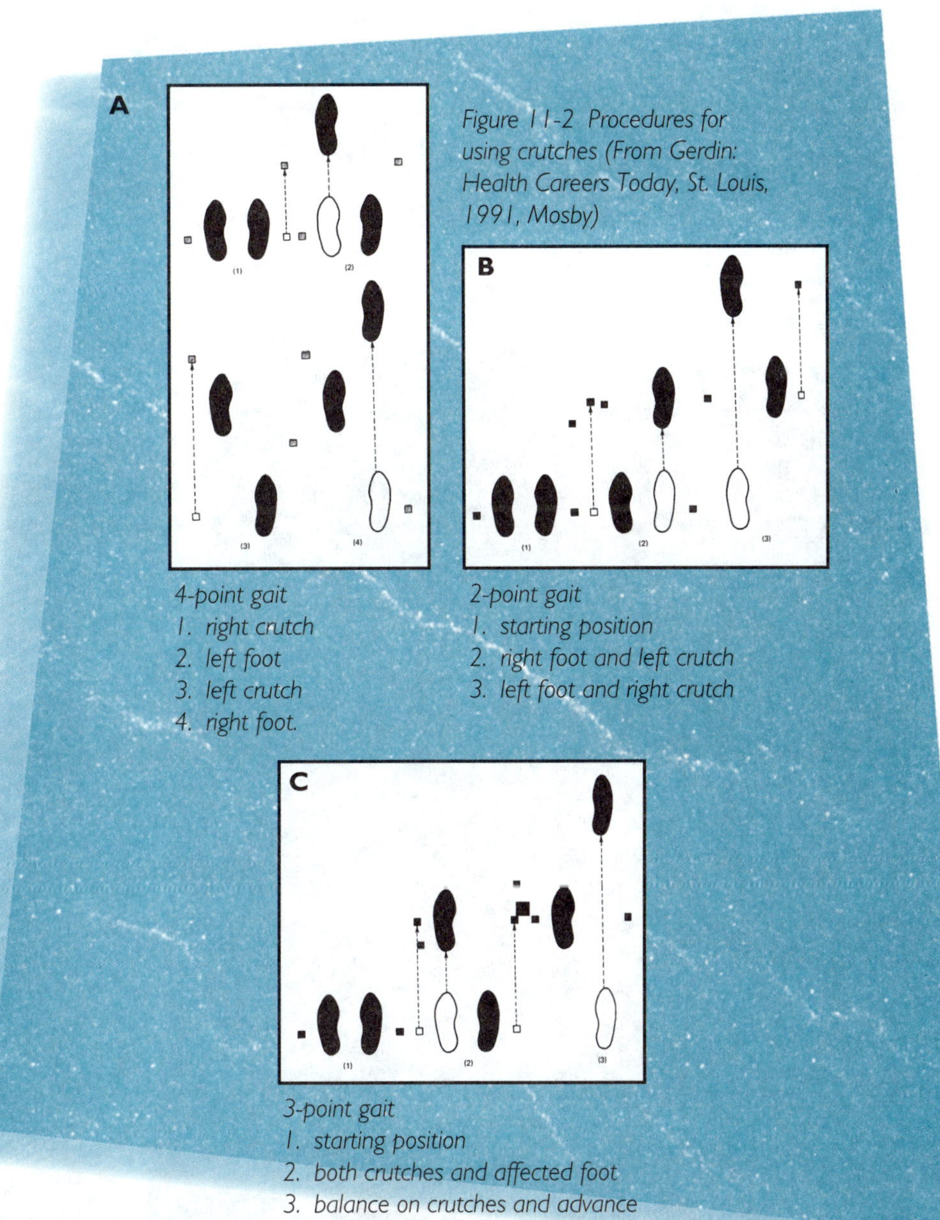

Figure 11-2 Procedures for using crutches (From Gerdin: Health Careers Today, St. Louis, 1991, Mosby)

4-point gait
1. right crutch
2. left foot
3. left crutch
4. right foot.

2-point gait
1. starting position
2. right foot and left crutch
3. left foot and right crutch

3-point gait
1. starting position
2. both crutches and affected foot
3. balance on crutches and advance unaffected foot

Multiple Choice

From the options listed under each question or statement, select the correct answer or answers. Write the corresponding letter or letters in the answer space.

1. The purpose of physical therapy is to: _______
   a. relieve pain
   b. increase circulation
   c. build strength
   d. restore and improve muscular function
   e. increase the range of motion or mobility of a joint
   f. all of the above

2. Safe body mechanics include all of the following principles except: _______
   a. proper body alignment
   b. balance
   c. coordination
   d. movement

3. When sitting straight in a chair: _______
   a. add support by placing a pillow behind your lower back
   b. elevate feet on a low stool
   c. cross legs and alternate every 15 minutes
   d. none of the above

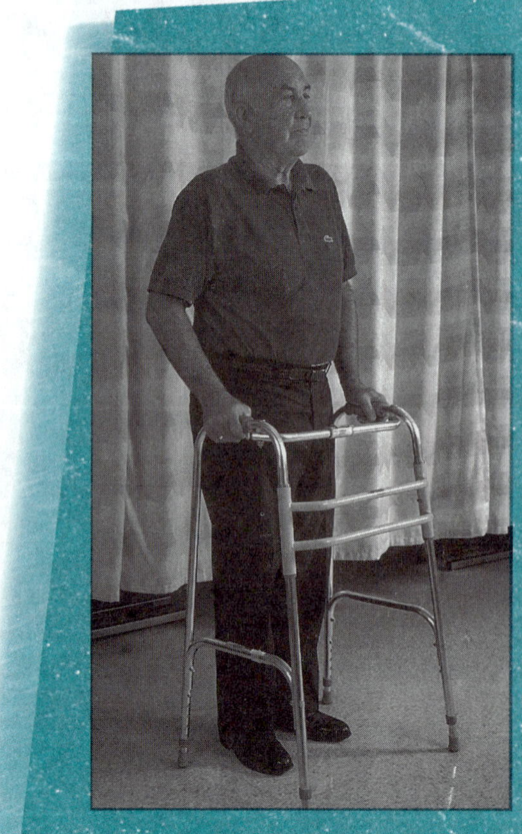

Figure 11-3 Patient using a stationary walker. Note the height of the walker and the position of the patient's arms.

4. Thermotherapy is used to: _______
   a. relieve pain
   b. promote muscle relaxation and reduce spasms
   c. increase circulation to an area
   d. relieve congestion and swelling
   e. speed up the inflammatory process and promote drainage
   f. all of the above

5. The purpose of a massage is to do all of the following except: _______
   a. increase circulation
   b. increase strength
   c. relieve spasms
   d. reduce pain
   e. all of the above

6. _______ exercises require that the patient perform all exercise motions without assistance.
   a. range of motion
   b. passive
   c. active
   d. aided

7. Dry heat may be applied using: _______
   a. heat lamp
   b. heating pad
   c. hot water bottle
   d. chemical hot pack
   e. a & b
   f. c & d
   g. all of the above

8. Moist heat applications frequently used include all of the following except: _______
   a. heating pad
   b. hot soaks
   c. hot compresses
   d. hot packs

9. Which type crutch gait is used to assist the person who can bear partial weight on both legs and can move both legs separately? _______
   a. two-point gait
   b. three-point gait
   c. four-point gait

10. When exercises are performed, the patient applies pressure or moves a part, and the assistant applies resistance to the movement: _______
    a. passive
    b. active
    c. passive resistive
    d. active resistive

11. Cryotherapy is used to: _______
    a. prevent edema or swelling
    b. relieve pain or tenderness
    c. reduce inflammation and pus formation
    d. control bleeding and reduce body temperature
    e. a, c, and d
    f. all of the above

12. Aided exercises are: _______
    a. performed when the patient moves without assistance
    b. exercises with patients whose muscles are too weak to move totally by their own strength
    c. exercises performed when the patient applies pressure or moves a part
    d. exercises performed by another person or outside force

13. Moist cold applications include all of the following except: _______
    a. cold compresses
    b. chemical cold packs
    c. ice massage
    d. alcohol sponge baths

14. Dry, cold applications frequently used include: _______
    a. ice bags
    b. ice collars
    c. chemical cold packs
    d. a, b, and c
    e. a and c
    f. none of the above

True or False

Determine whether each of the following statements is true or false. Check the box marked T or F at the left of the statement.

T   F

☐ ☐   1. Only a physical therapist can give physical therapy treatments.

☐ ☐   2. The basics of good body mechanics hinge on good posture.

☐ ☐   3. Pulling is easier on your back than pushing.

☐ ☐   4. Placing something under the feet will reduce back tension when sitting for long periods of time.

☐ ☐   5. It is important for a medical assistant to learn some of the basics of physical therapy.

☐ ☐   6. Superficial heat treatments can be given with local dry or moist heat applications.

☐ ☐   7. The three-point gait is used when the patient can support his full weight on one leg and partial weight on the other leg.

☐ ☐   8. Use the spine as a series of separate vertebrae.

☐ ☐   9. Bending your knees so that you use the large leg muscles during lifting is recommended.

☐ ☐   10. To relieve strain on the lower back, lift the foot to return the spine to its natural curve.

☐ ☐   11. Abduction is when a body part is brought toward the midline.

☐ ☐   12. When sitting or standing, keep your spine balanced.

☐ ☐   13. Therapeutic exercise is designed to correct a physical deformity.

☐ ☐   14. Hold items at arm's length and maintain a firm grip on the item.

☐ ☐   15. Twist or pivot when lifting items to prevent back injury.

☐ ☐   16. Pronation is movement of the arm to have the palm facing upward.

☐ ☐   17. The shoulder blades are called clavicles.

☐ ☐   18. Acceptable water temperatures range from 105 to 115 degrees F. for patient two years or older.

☐ ☐   19. Canes may be recommended to the patient with poor balance.

☐ ☐   20. Body mechanics refers to how you use your body when lifting, pushing, or even lying down.

Word Puzzle

Fill in each line with a word related to physical therapy from the video or workbook that fits the definitions below. When the puzzle is completed, the highlighted vertical column will answer the question: "What is the treatment of disease that uses dry and moist heat application?"

ACROSS

1. patient performs all exercise motions without assistance
2. _______ point gait used when the patient can support full weight on one leg and partial weight on the other
3. exercise performed by another person without voluntary assistance from the patient
4. palm facing down
5. hands or feet can be flexed and bent backward
6. palm facing upward
7. how you use your body when you perform physical actions
8. bent
9. the leg may be _______ or externally rotated
10. a part moved away from the midline of the body
11. shoulder blades
12. treatment with cold

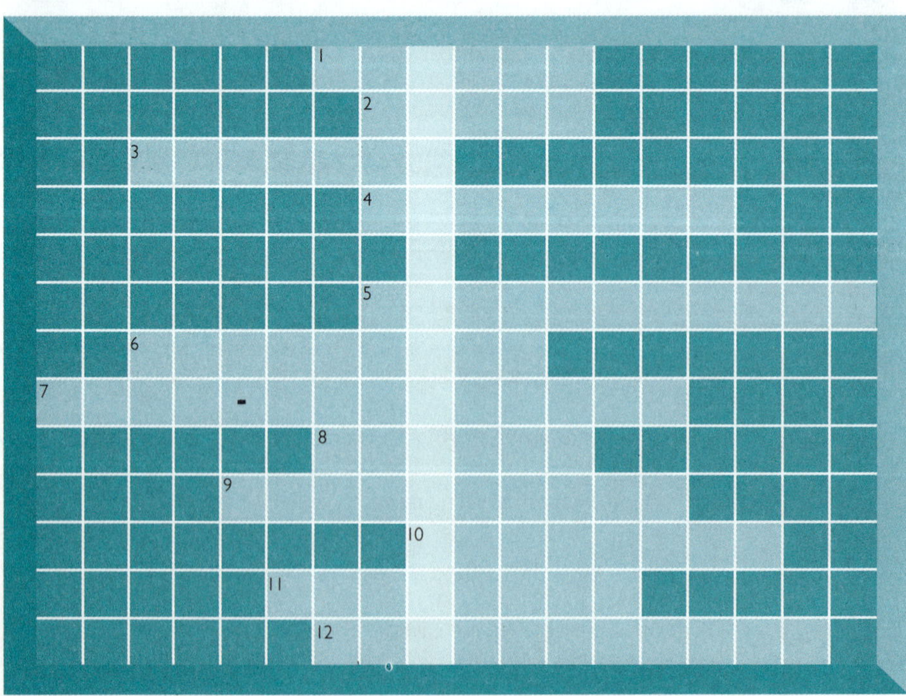

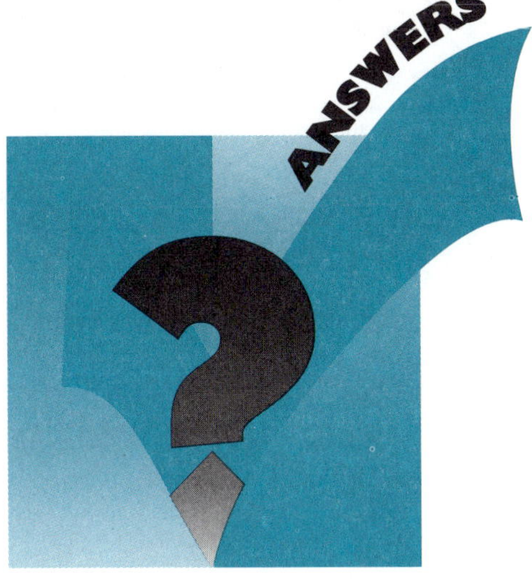

Vocabulary

1. o	5. e	9. c	13. j	17. q
2. i	6. l	10. d	14. g	18. h
3. k	7. b	11. m	15. n	19. t
4. f	8. r	12. a	16. p	20. s

Student Activities

1 3. Answers may vary.

Discussion Topics

1. Answer may vary.

2. *MVA* - motor vehicle accident

   Disposition - plan or discharge

   Myofascial strain - strain of the muscle and fascia

   AROM - active range of motion

   Objective - signs and symptoms found on examination

   ADL - activities of daily living

Review and Rationale

1. Standing with feet apart and one foot slightly in front of the other provides a stable, wide base of support.

2. When you need to stand for a long period of time with little movement, place one foot on a low stool to help keep your spine in balance; occasionally alternate feet.

3. To prevent burns while using a heat lamp, keep it at least two to four feet away from the skin depending on the type and intensity of the lamp.

4. To prevent injury caused by burns, always place an electric heating pad in a protective covering such as a pillow case before applying it to a dry area.

5. When performing cryotherapy, check the patient periodically for changes such as a decrease or increase in swelling or redness on the area, or a decrease or increase in pain.

6. Always cover the thermotherapy pack with a cloth before applying it to the patient's skin to prevent the skin from burning.

7. By having the patient hold the cane on the opposite side of the weakness, the cane supports and takes the weight off the weak leg.

8. The patient should never lie on the pad because burns could result.

9. Place additional toweling over the ice to reduce the melting rate.

10. When showing the patient his prescribed gait, be sure to reinforce two important principles of walking with crutches: Always look straight ahead to prevent falling. Always rest your weight on the palms of the hands, not on the axillary bars of the crutch. This gives a more even distribution of weight and prevents muscle fatigue.

11. When you as a medical assistant teach the patient any exercises, you must explain the reasons for the exercise, and then assess the patient's exercise capabilities. This will prevent the patient from injury. Thoroughly demonstrate each exercise, and then ask the patient to perform the exercises in the office until the patient fully understands the motion involved.

12. Only filling a hot water bottle one-half full and expelling the air before putting the top on allows the hot water bottle to be more pliable.

13. The type of assistive device used depends on the patient's disability.

14. When transferring a patient to and from the wheelchair, keep in mind safety precautions and proper body mechanics to prevent injury to yourself and/or the patient.

15. Maintain the temperature as much as possible through thermotherapy by removing some of the solution every five minutes or so and adding more hot solution.

Multiple Choice

1. f	4. f	7. g	10. d	13. b
2. c	5. b	8. a	11. e	14. d
3. a	6. c	9. c	12. b	

True or False

1. F	5. T	9. T	13. T	17. F
2. T	6. T	10. T	14. F	18. F
3. F	7. T	11. F	15. F	19. F
4. T	8. F	12. T	16. F	20. T

Word Puzzle

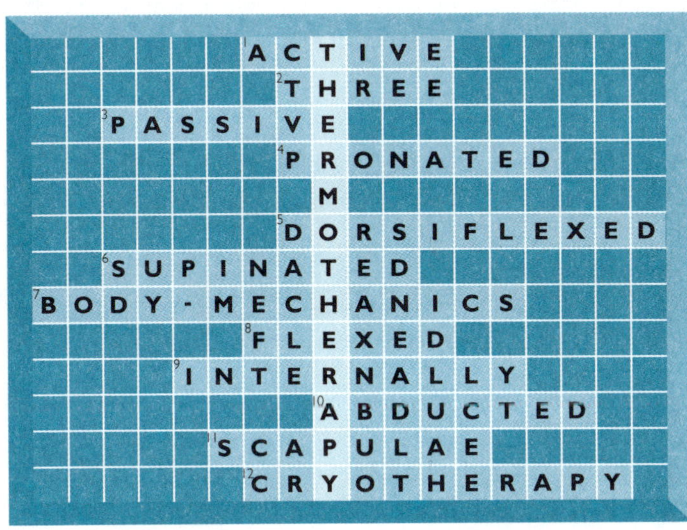

HISTORICAL HIGHLIGHTS

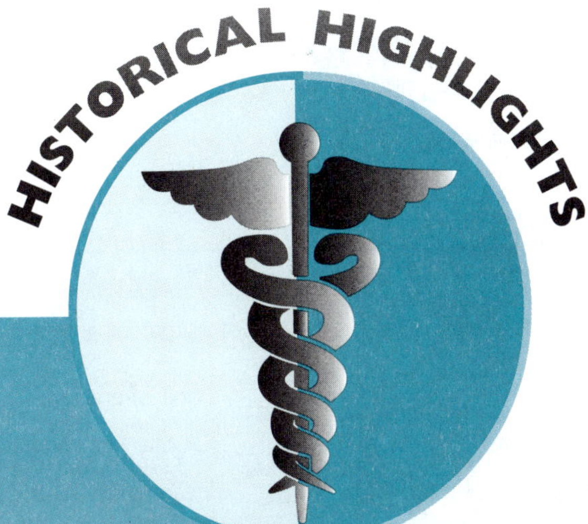

Tools to treat man have been used perhaps as early as 10,000 B.C. Crude in design, heavy in weight, beautiful in ornamentation, tools assisted the physician to perform cutting and repairing wounds. Through the ages, these tools have evolved into the precision surgical instruments of today.

Joseph Lister stated that success is attention to detail. This is the essence of the state of the art as practiced in all of the medical specialties. Handling and preparing sophisticated instruments and equipment for a procedure is no exception.

The addition of electrical power to provide light or permit the functioning of medical equipment is an additional concern for the medical assistant who must be aware of and safeguard against the hazards of electrical shock while performing duties. Electrocardiogram electrodes should be placed as far away from the operative site as possible; needle electrodes should be avoided as they could transmit leakage currents into the body; and burns can occur at sites of ECG electrodes. The environment must be safe for both patients and personnel.

You will be required to administer electrocardiographic procedures either independently or as an assistant. As you develop familiarity with these procedures, your skill and confidence will increase, and your professionalism will be appreciated by your patients and the physician.

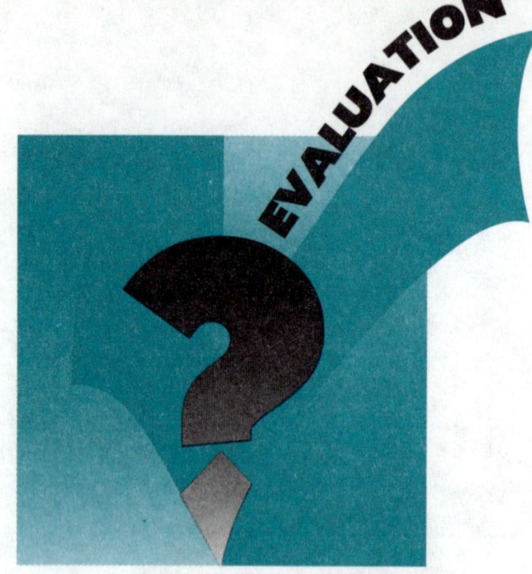

Vocabulary

Write the letter of each term on the line of its matching definition at the right.

a. electrolyte

b. somatic tremor

c. electrocardiograph

d. electrode

e. artifacts

f. ambulatory monitoring

g. AC

h. palpitations

i. electrocardiogram

j. joules

k. conductive jelly

l. skin rasp

m. Holter monitor

n. xiphoid process

o. syncope

p. CPR

q. sinoatrial node

r. arrhythmia

s. tachycardia

t. defibrillation

1. _______ a unit of energy

2. _______ voluntary or involuntary muscle movement

3. _______ "pacemaker" of the heart

4. _______ "fluttering" heartbeat

5. _______ abnormal rhythm of the heart

6. _______ unwanted activity on the ECG

7. _______ a record of the electrical activity of the heart

8. _______ rapid heart rate

9. _______ instrument used to record electrical activity of the heart

10. _______ ambulatory monitoring device to record continuous ECG activity

11. _______ continuous recording of the electrical activity of the patient's heart for 24-48 hours

12. _______ electrolyte

13. _______ device used to remove dead skin from electrode site

14. _______ sensors or small metal plates or disposable units

15. _______ losing consciousness

16. _______ point of the sternum

17. _______ gels, pastes, or flannel materials presaturated with solution used to improve conductivity of electricity

18. _______ alternating current

19. _______ high intensity electrical charge to the heart

20. _______ cardiopulmonary resuscitation

Student Activities

1. Research the various ECG equipment that offers features most required in a physician's office for routine electrocardiography. Compare features and costs and present your recommendations.

2. Based on Student Activity #1, invite a representative from the vendor of the ECG equipment to visit the classroom to demonstrate the equipment.

Discussion Topics

Case Study 1

The following case study illustrates cardiovascular disease in a patient being evaluated for cataract extraction and lens implantation. Define the medical terminology and discuss the impact of the patient's ECG.

HISTORY: The patient is a 91-year-old white female who is scheduled for outpatient left cataract extraction and lens implantation. She has bilateral cataracts and her vision is so poor now that she is unable to play bingo or read.

PAST MEDICAL HISTORY: She was hospitalized from 1/23/94 to 1/29/94 with the following diagnosis:

   a) Coronary atherosclerotic heart disease, hypertensive heart disease, valvular heart disease with aortic stenosis, congestive heart failure and left bundle branch block and resultant cardiac arrest; defibrillation was successful. Subsequent electrocar-

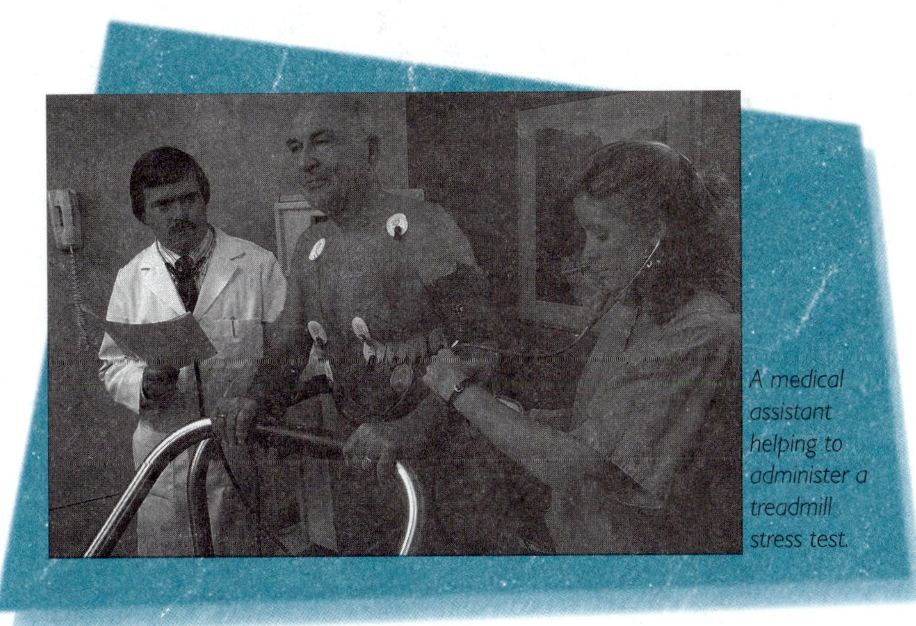

A medical assistant helping to administer a treadmill stress test.

diographic studies revealed myocardial infarction with extensive damage of myocardium and continued arrhythmia.

b) History of hypertension.

c) Borderline elevated TSH.

d) S/P bilateral mastectomies for carcinoma.

ELECTROCARDIOGRAPHY WITH INTERPRETATION Sinus rhythm, rate 80; PR: 24; QRS:.09. There is left axis deviation. There are minimal nonspecific ST-T wave changes. Q waves in the inferior leads compatible with, although not diagnostic of prior inferior wall myocardial infarction. No change from previous study.

Case Study 2

This is the first time Mrs. Murez has had an ECG performed. She does not speak English fluently and needs additional assistance due to a fractured right forearm immobilized in a cast. She is quite nervous and is reluctant to undress. Explain how you will prepare this patient for the ECG.

Case Study 3

During preparation of Mr. Peatro for routine ECG, you determine an elevated blood pressure and irregular heart rate. What precautions should be observed?

Review and Rationale

Answer the following questions in the space provided.

1. Why should you develop skills in electrocardiography?

____

____

____

2. Why does a disturbance in the cardiac cycle cause a change in the normal electrical forces needed to maintain the heart beat?

____

____

____

3. Why does the physician observe and measure the baseline, waves, and time intervals on the ECG?

____

____

____

4. Why are there standard techniques for ECG performance?

____

____

____

5. Why should you check the machine to determine if it is set to record according to the universal measurement?

____

____

____

6. Why should the electrocardiograph room be prepared so that other machinery, wires, and cords are as far away as possible from the ECG machine?

____

____

____

7. Why should the patient remove any jewelry prior to having the ECG performed?

____

____

____

8. Why should the patient remove thick stockings?

____

____

____

9. Why should you place the ECG electrode on a flat, fleshy surface of each extremity?

____

____

____

10. Why apply the electrodes with the tab pointing in the direction of the lead-wire?

____

____

____

11. Why do you place all six chest electrodes on at the same time when using a three channel ECG system?

____

____

____

12. Why do you place the chest lead in an out of the way position when recording the individual limb leads?

____

____

____

13. Why arrange the lead-wires to follow the contours of the body?

____

____

____

14. Why are you expected to understand the causes of artifacts?

____

____

____

15. Why does Holter monitoring record electrical activity of the heart during unrestricted activity, rest, and sleep over a 24 to 48 hour period?

____

____

____

16. Why does the patient keep a diary of his/her activities, noting the time of day during Holter monitoring?

____

____

____

17. Why should you be careful to avoid pressing the center or "gel cap" of the electrode?

____

____

____

18. Why shave the patient's chest in areas where the electrodes will be placed?

____

____

____

Performance Test

In a skills laboratory, a simulation of a job-like environment, the medical assistant student must demonstrate skill and knowledge in performing the following procedures without reference to source materials. Time limits for the performance of each procedure are to be assigned by the instructor.

1. Prepare the patient for an electrocardiogram.

2. Locate the six chest lead positions on three individuals. Figure 12-1, diagram of a twelve-lead ECG, clearly demonstrates the 6 chest lead positions.

3. Apply the electrodes and lead-wires.

4. Record the ECGs.

5. Mount the results.

6. Correctly care for the equipment after use.

You are to perform the above activities with 100% accuracy 90% of the time (9 out of 10

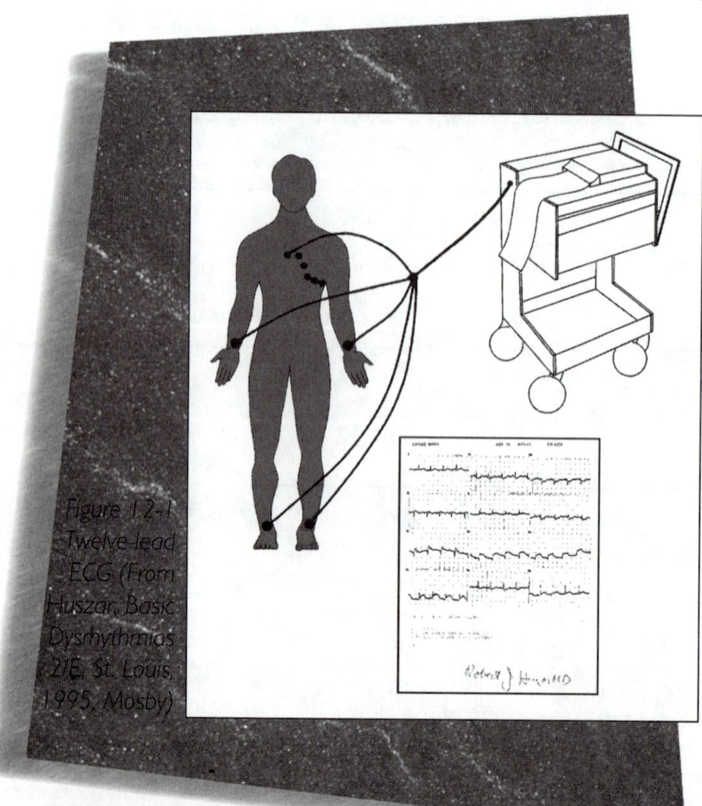

Figure 12-1 Twelve-lead ECG (From Huszar, Basic Dysrhythmias 2/E, St. Louis, 1995, Mosby)

Performance Checklist

DIRECTIONS: The following checklist will be used to evaluate your performance of each procedure.

Checklist 12-1: Obtaining an Electrocardiogram

Checklist	S or NA	U	NO	Comment
1. Assemble equipment needed to perform an ECG				
2. Prepare room and equipment.				
3. Prepare patient.				
a. Explain nature and purpose of ECG.				
b. Ask patient to remove shoes and all clothing above the waist and put on patient gown with opening in the front. Ask patient to remove any jewelry.				
c. Place patient in supine position with small pillow under the head.				
d. Ask patient not to move, talk, or chew gum.				
e. Check that all extremities are well supported and that legs are not touching one another.				
f. Place drape over arms and lower part of legs.				
g. Ask patient if he has any questions regarding the procedure.				
4. Before placing electrodes, remove lotion or oil from skin surface of the electrode sites with alcohol sponges.				
5. Locate the 6 chest lead positions and mark with a felt tip pen.				
6. Using electrolyte gel, paste, or pad, place the electrode on selected site. (Disposable tab diagnostic ECG electrodes may be used.)				
7. Attach electrode and appropriate lead-wire with the tab pointing in the direction of the lead-wire tension.				

*S or NA = satisfactory or not applicable; U = unsatisfactory; NO = not observed

Continued on next page

Continued from previous page

Checklist 12-1: Obtaining an Electrocardiogram

Checklist	S or NA	U	NO	Comment
8. Attach chest electrodes.				
a. If using a three channel ECG system, all six chest electrodes must be placed on at the same time.				
b. If using a one channel system, the recordings for each limb lead and chest lead are recorded separately.				
c. Preserve patient modesty and comfort at all times.				
9. Check that each lead-wire is correctly attached to the appropriate electrode.				
10. Plug the patient cable into the cable jack on the machine.				
11. Enter the patient information on the keyboard.				
12. Select auto ECG format. Push auto.				
13. Ask patient to remain still until the "auto complete" message appears.				
14. After completing the ECG tracing and determining it is of good quality, disconnect the patient from the machine.				
15. Disconnect the lead-wires and unfasten and remove the electrodes for the patient.				
16. Wipe off any electrolyte gel or paste and pen marks from the skin.				
17. Assist the patient to dress as needed and provide any further instruction or information as indicated.				
18. If ECG system is not automatic, label all ECG recordings and mount properly (record patient's name, date, and your initials).				
19. Clean the equipment and return it to proper storage area.				
20. Wash your hands.				
21. Record the procedure.				

**S or NA = satisfactory or not applicable; U = unsatisfactory; NO = not observed*

Multiple Choice

From the options listed under each question or statement, select the correct answer or answers. Write the corresponding letter or letters in the answer space.

1. Name the three types of artifacts on electrocardiograms: ________
    a. muscle movement, wandering baseline, alternating current interference
    b. somatic tremor, jagged peaks, irregular height
    c. AC interference, somatic tremor, wandering baseline
    d. any of the above

2. What is the term for voluntary or involuntary movement? ________
    a. artifacts
    b. somatic tremor
    c. Parkinson disease
    d. parkinsonism

3. Which of the following does not contribute to wandering baseline artifacts? ________
    a. electrodes applied too tightly or loosely
    b. corroded or dirty electrodes
    c. presence of other electrical equipment in the room
    d. too little or poor quality electrolyte gel on the electrodes

4. A series of small, regular peaks or spiked lines on the electrocardiogram is called: ________
    a. static electricity
    b. joules interference
    c. wandering baseline
    d. alternating current artifacts

5. Which of the following will minimize or eliminate AC interference? ________
    a. straightening lead-wires to follow body contour
    b. move the patient table away from the wall
    c. remove x-ray equipment from room
    d. all of the above

6. Which of the following data is not essential documentation for electrocardiography? ________
    a. name, address, age
    b. drugs patient is taking
    c. sex and date of ECG
    d. blood pressure, height, and weight
    e. all of the above

7. What is Holter monitoring? _______
   a. Phone-A-Gram
   b. ambulatory cardiac monitoring
   c. defibrillation
   d. automatic electrocardiography

8. Which of the following is used to remove dead skin from the electrode site in preparation for application of the electrode? _______
   a. a razor
   b. skin rasp
   c. nonallergenic adhesive tape
   d. alcohol sponges

9. Applying pressure to the gel cap will cause: _______
   a. a chemical reaction to the gel producing heat
   b. the electrode to properly adhere to the electrode site
   c. the conductive gel to ooze out onto the adhesive ring
   d. minimizing of AC artifacts

10. What type of information should be recorded in the patient diary? _______
    a. pain or discomfort
    b. taking medication
    c. under stress
    d. all of the above

True or False

Determine whether each of the following statements is true or false. Check the box marked T or F at the left of the statement.

T F

☐ ☐ 1. Artifacts are defects on an ECG.

☐ ☐ 2. Somatic tremor produces a wandering baseline.

☐ ☐ 3. Dirty electrodes causes alternating current interference.

☐ ☐ 4. Straightening and positioning lead-wires to follow body contour will minimize AC interference.

☐ ☐ 5. All ECG machines generate page-size printouts.

☐ ☐ 6. Ambulatory cardiac monitoring is also referred to as Holter monitoring.

T   F

7. Electrocardiography uses advanced electro-medical technology to give precise diagnostic information about a patient's heart.

8. A standard twelve-lead ECG has four bipolar limb leads.

9. The electrolyte is a small metal plate.

10. When using a three channel ECG system, the six chest electrodes are placed on one at a time.

11. You place all six chest electrodes on at the same time when using a three channel ECG system because in the three channel system the limb leads and chest leads are recorded simultaneously, giving you the twelve views of the heart.

12. The chest lead must be placed in a position where it will not cause artifacts while recording individual limb leads.

13. Arrange the lead-wires to follow the contours of the body. To minimize the possibility of AC artifacts, no strain should be placed on the electrodes.

14. You will be expected to understand the causes of artifacts so you can eliminate or minimize them.

15. Holter monitoring is done to detect cardiac rhythm disturbances and correlate them with patient symptoms of chest pain, palpitations, dizziness, syncope, or fatigue.

16. While wearing the monitor, the patient keeps a diary of his/her activities, noting the time of day. Special notation is made of stressful or significant events, or of cardiac symptoms.

17. Press the center or "gel cap" of the electrode to release the conductive gel onto the adhesive ring.

18. Shaving the patient's chest in areas where the electrodes will be placed is optional.

Word Puzzle

Fill in each line with a word related to electrocardiography from the video or workbook that fits the definitions below. When the puzzle is completed, the highlighted vertical column will answer the question: "What test uses advanced electro-medical technology to give precise diagnostic information about a patient's heart?"

ACROSS

____________ 1. sensors or small metal plates or disposable units

____________ 2. gels, pastes, or flannel materials presaturated with solution used to improve conductivity of electricity

____________ 3. electrolyte

____________ 4. cardiopulmonary resuscitation

____________ 5/6. voluntary or involuntary muscle movement

____________ 7. a unit of energy (joule)

____________ 8. rapid heart rate

____________ 9. unwanted activity on the ECG

____________ 10. high intensity, electrical charge to the heart

____________ 11. not reusable, one-time service

____________ 12. "fluttering" heartbeat

____________ 13. "pacemaker" of the heart

____________ 14. instrument used to record electrical activity of the heart

____________ 15. ambulatory monitoring device to record continuous ECG activity

____________ 16. device used to remove dead skin from electrode site

____________ 17. point of the sternum

____________ 18. abnormal rhythm of the heart

____________ 19. losing consciousness

DOWN

____________ 20. What test uses advanced electro-medical technology to give precise diagnostic information about a patient's heart?

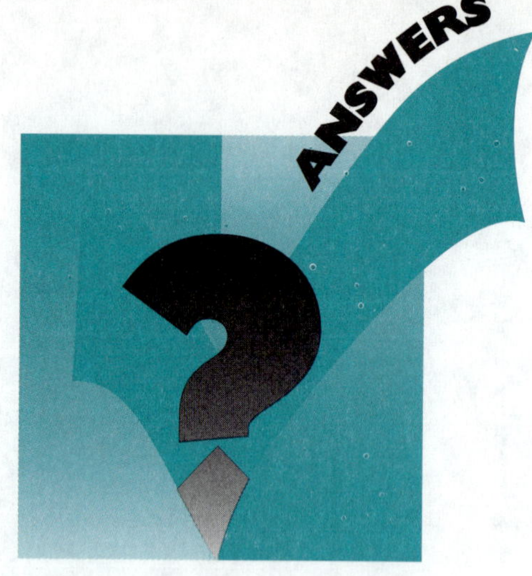

Vocabulary

1. j	5. r	9. c	13. l	17. a
2. b	6. e	10. f	14. d	18. g
3. q	7. i	11. m	15. o	19. t
4. h	8. s	12. k	16. n	20. p

Student Activities

1–2. Answers may vary.

Discussion Topics

Case Study 1: Answers may vary. Be sure you understand all medical terminology. Consult a medical dictionary to confirm pronunciation and definitions.

Case Study 2: Answers may vary.

Case Study 3: Answers may vary, but should include immediate notification of the physician.

Review and Rationale

1. The more knowledge and skills you develop in electrocardiography, the more effective you will be as a medical assistant.

2. Any disturbance in the cardiac cycle will cause a change in the normal electrical forces needed to maintain the heart beat. This disturbance may produce an arrhythmia, which is an irregularity in the heart rhythm.

3. The physician can analyze and interpret the rate, rhythm, and conduction of the heart by observing and measuring the baseline, waves, and time intervals.

4. Standard techniques have been adapted so that an ECG recording may be interpreted anywhere in the world.

5. Check the ECG machine to determine if it is set to record according to the universal measurement before recording an ECG tracing to assure accuracy and consistency.

6. This helps prevent electrical defects, known as artifacts, from appearing on the ECG tracing; artifacts make it difficult for the physician to interpret the ECG.

7. Jewelry may interfere with electrode placement.

8. Thick stockings should be removed as they will cause artifacts on the tracing.

9. Place the electrode on a flat, fleshy surface of each extremity to minimize the chance of artifacts.

10. Applying the electrodes with the tab pointing in the direction of the lead-wire will minimize tension on it.

11. You place all six chest electrodes at the same time because in the three channel system the limb leads are recorded simultaneously giving you the twelve views of the heart.

12. The chest lead is not needed while recording the individual limb leads, and must be placed in a position where it will not cause artifacts.

13. Arrange the lead-wires to follow the contours of the body to minimize the possibility of AC artifacts so no strain is placed on the electrodes.

14. You will be expected to understand the causes of artifacts, such as machinery or electrical device interference, and how they can be eliminated or minimized.

15. Holter monitoring is done to detect cardiac rhythm disturbances and correlate them with patient symptoms of chest pain, palpitations, dizziness, syncope, or fatigue over a prolonged period of time.

16. The patient keeps a diary of his/her activities, noting the time of day with special notation of stressful or significant events, or of cardiac symptoms. The activities are correlated with the ECG tracing to see if the abnormal rhythm is present at the same time as the symptom.

17. Pressing the center or "gel cap" of the electrode may cause conductive gel to ooze out onto the adhesive ring.

18. Shaving the patient's chest in the areas where the electrodes will be placed prepares the skin for receiving the electrode without interference.

Multiple Choice

1. a.	3. c	5. d	7. b	9. c
2. b	4. d	6. e	8. b	10. d

True or False

1. T	5. F	9. F	13. T	17. F
2. F	6. T	10. T	14. T	18. F
3. F	7. T	11. T	15. T	
4. T	8. T	12. T	16. T	

Word Puzzle

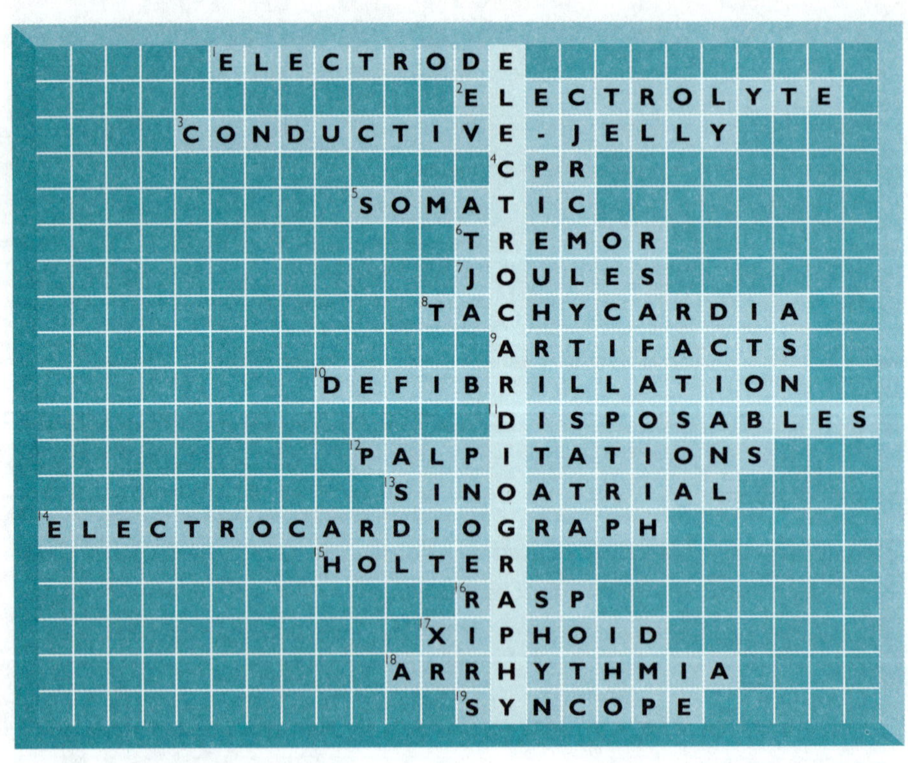